PRINCIPLES OF HUMAN MOVEMENT CONTROL AND DYSFUNCTION

Xu-Feng Huang, MD, PhD, DSc

Professor of Medical Science

School of Medical, Indigenous, and Health Sciences

The University of Wollongong
Australia
2022

Ashahi-Maple

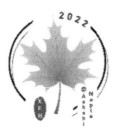

Copyright @ Ashahi-Maple

The copy right of the author Xu-Feng Huang has been asserted by him in accordance with the Copyright Amendment (Moral Right) Act 2000.

All rights reserved. This book is protected by copyright. No part of this publication may be reproduced, copied, scanned, stored in or introduced into a retrieval system, or transmitted, in any form or by any means, without the prior written permission of both the copyright owner and publisher of this book apart from any use as permitted under the Copyright Act 1968.

National Library of Australia Cataloguing-in-Publication Data is available.

First published in Australia in 2022
by Ashahi-Maple©, Inc.

ISBN 978-0-6454760-3-3

TO MY FAMILY

Preface

Who is this book for? This reference book serves as a comprehensive guide for understanding the principles of human movement control and dysfunction. It is an essential resource for students of exercise and sport science, exercise physiologists, chiropractors, fitness trainers, healthcare professionals, and researchers alike. With its in-depth coverage of the topic, the book is designed to provide readers with the necessary knowledge and skills to excel in their respective fields

This book aims to: (1) explain the mechanism of human movement control, (2) describe the cause of movement abnormalities, and (3) develop the ability to read, understand, and evaluate current professional literature.

Contents: This book has twelve chapters covering the theories of voluntary movement, posture and balance, motor learning, cortex, basal ganglia and spinal control, neuromuscular junction, muscle and their respective abnormalities and examinations. At the end, it describe common upper limb, lower limb and vertebral injuries followed by future research directions in motor control.

Expectations: Readers will be able to explain both the mechanisms of voluntary movement controls and dysfunctions, allowing them to apply this knowledge to their professional practice.

Professor Xu-Feng Huang, MD, PhD, DSc

CONTENTS

Chapter 1: Introduction to movement control 1

   Human brain 3

      Broadmann's Brain Map 3

      Primary Motor Map 5

      Cortical homunculus 10

      Somatosensory cortex 13

      Cortical-cortical connections 15

   Motor Control Theories 17

      Hierarchical, system, and ecological models 17

      Somatic motor control hierarchy 20

   Sensorimotor Integration 23

Chapter 2: Motor learning 27

   Introduction to motor learning 28

      Basic concept of motor learning 28

      Types of motor skills 29

      Stages of motor learning 30

      Motor skill acquisition and retention 32

Feedback 33

    Feedback in motor learning 33

    Feedback be used to improve motor skills 35

    Intrinsic feedback of motor learning 36

    Extrinsic feedback of motor learning 38

Practice 39

    The role of practice 39

    Practice impact skill acquisition and retention 41

    What is the deliberate practice? 42

    Effectiveness of practice 44

Environmental factors 46

    Equipment 46

    Coaching 46

    Social support 47

Special populations 47

    Motor learning in children, older adults and individuals with disabilities 47

    Motor development, control, and rehabilitation in specific populations 49

Applications 50

    Real-world settings 50

    Examples 54

    Motor control and sport performance 55

    Motor control in older people 57

Chapter 3: Cortex 59

  Somatomotor Cortex and Voluntary Movement 59

    Cortical Motor Neural Mapping 59

    Presetting, Precision, and Orientation 67

    Spike-Triggered Averaging 73

    Plasticity of the Cortical Motor Map 74

  Association Motor Cortex 77

    Anatomy 79

    Connections of the Association Motor Cortex 85

    Stimulation of the Association Motor Cortex 86

    Association Motor Cortical Map 87

    Externally Guided Movement 88

    Internally guided movement 90

    Premovement Potential 95

  Brain injury 97

    Human motor dysfunction 98

    Brain Trauma 100

    Cerebellar Motor Syndrome 107

    Cerebral Injury 108

    Primary Motor Cortex Lesions 111

    Cortex Abnormality 112

    Cerebellum 118

    Epilepsy 119

Chapter 4: Basal Ganglia and Movement Quality 120

    Structure and function 121

        Anatomy 121

        Function 124

    Pathways 133

        Basal Ganglia Motor Regulatory Pathways 133

    Abnormalities 136

        Movement quality alterations 136

        Parkinson's Disease 150

        Huntington's Disease 162

        Ballism 165

        Stroke 168

        Internal Capsule Lesion 169

Chapter 5: Spinal Cord Regulates Motor Function 174

- Spinal Cord 175
- Upper Motor Neurons 176
- Lower Motor Neurons 177
  - Alpha Motor Neuron 181
  - What inputs can influence alpha motor neuron? 183
  - Motor unit 184
  - Gamma Motor Neuron 190
  - Spinal Interneurons 192
  - Sensory Inputs related to motor control 194
  - Sensory nerve regulates motor function 196
  - Superficial sensation influences motor control 199
- Muscles 212
  - Muscle spindle 212
  - Intrafusal muscle fibers 213
  - Extrafusal muscle fibers 214
  - Sustained voluntary muscle contraction 215
  - Golgi Tendon Organ 216
- Neuromuscular Control 218
- Motor Reflex 220
  - Golgi tendon reflex 220

Stretch Reflex 222

Clasp-Knife Reflex 226

Reciprocal Inhibition Reflex 227

Polysynaptic flexor reflex 231

Gag reflex 234

Crossed Extensor Reflex 235

Generation of spinal motor programs for walking 238

What is an automated movement? 242

What is nerve-induced plasticity of muscle fibers? 246

Electromyography 247

Nerve conduction velocity test 248

Spinal Cord Injury 251

The upper and lower motor injuries 252

Paraplegia 253

Quadriplegia 254

Spinal cord injury causes sensation Loss 255

Upper Motor Neuron Syndrome 256

Lower Motor Neuron Syndrome 257

Pyramidal Signs 258

Chapter 6: Body Posture, Arm Reaching, and Fine Movement ... 264

Head and neck movements 265
    Vestibulo-ocular reflex 267
    Cervicocollic reflex 269
    Cranial nerves control head muscles 269
    Somatomotor cortex controls head and neck muscles 271
    Head and neck muscle groups and motor dysfunction 273
    Upper motor neurons control the head and neck muscles .. 274
    Lower motor neurons control the head and neck muscles . 275
    Vestibulospinal tract controls posture and head movements
    277
    Tectospinal tract controls head movements 280
    Orienting reflex 281
    How does the reticulospinal tract control head muscles? ... 282
Body posture and balance regulation 284
    Trunk movements 284
    Lateral corticospinal tract controls movements? 286
    The reflex loop maintains body posture 288
    The reflex loop maintains body balance 290
    Clinical examination of three input integrity for body balance control 293
    Three Steps of Rescue Reactions 294

Vestibular System regulates body balance 295

Cerebellar Ataxia 303

Arm Reaching 305

Fine movements 307

Chapter 7: Neuromuscular Junction Diseases 310

Neuromuscular Junction Structure 310

Synaptic Cleft 311

Motor End Plate 313

Transmission Pathway 313

Types of Acetylcholine Receptors 314

Neuromuscular Junction Disease 315

Myasthenia Gravis 317

Nerve Agents 319

Chapter 8: Skeletal muscle 321

Introduction 323

Histology 323

Skeletal muscle types 325

Muscles mainly made of type I muscles 326

Muscles mainly made of type II muscles 327

Molecular Basis of Muscle Contraction 328

Nutrition requirements for types I and type II muscles 330

Exercises influence muscle fiber types 331

Neuron or muscle changes first when we age 332

Muscle dysfunction 333

Muscle Weakness 334

Muscle weakness caused by upper motor neuron lesion 334

Muscle weakness caused by lower motor neuron injury 336

Muscle weakness and myopathy 337

Neurogenic muscle weakness 338

Myopathy 339

Duchenne Muscle Dystrophy 341

Myotonic dystrophy 343

Metabolic Myopathy 345

Polymyositis 346

Alcohol-Induced Myopathy 347

Viral Myalgia 348

Endocrine Myopathy 348

Muscle Tone Alteration 350

Muscle Examinations 351

Testing of voluntary muscle power 352

- Indirect Testing of Muscle Power 353
- Functional test and indirect test of muscle power 355
- Fasciculation 358
- Cogwheel rigidity 360

Chapter 9: Upper Limb Motor Dysfunction 362

- Nerve injury 363
  - Spinal nerves and motor dysfunction 364
  - Cranial Nerves and motor dysfunction 365
  - Brachial Plexus Injuries 366
  - Injuries to the supraclavicular part of the brachial plexus .. 367
  - Axillary Nerve Injury 371
  - Long Thoracic Nerve Injury 372
  - Median Nerve Injury 373
  - Radial Nerve Injury 374
  - Ulnar Nerve Injury 376
- Joint injury 379
  - Joint 380
  - Fibrous, cartilaginous, and synovial joints 380
  - Structures of Synovial Joint 382
  - Movements of the Joints 383

Joint dislocation 384

Clinical manifestations of joint injury 385

General Pathology of Joint Dislocation 386

Treatment of Joint Dislocation 386

General Pathology of Joint Dislocation 387

Shoulder joint dislocation 388

Anterior dislocation of the shoulder joint 389

Posterior dislocation of the shoulder joint 390

Complications of shoulder joint dislocation 390

Acromioclavicular Joint dislocation 392

Elbow Joint Dislocation 393

Bone fracture 394

Soft tissue damage 395

Fracture of the Olecranon 396

Fracture of the distal end of the radius 397

Fracture of the distal end of the radius 397

Impacted fracture of the humerus surgical neck 399

Transverse fracture of the body of the humerus 400

Transverse fracture of the body of the humerus 401

Fracture of the Scaphoid Bone 402

- Snuffbox 403
- Mallet or Baseball Finger 403
- Bursitis 404
  - Subacromial Bursitis 405
  - Student's elbow 406
  - Tennis elbow 407
  - Carpal Tunnel Syndrome 408
  - Raynaud's Phenomenon 409

Chapter 10 Lower Limb Motor Dysfunction 411

- Hip region 411
  - Hip joint movement 412
  - Sciatic nerve injury 413
  - Hip Joint Dislocation 414
  - Fracture of the Neck of the Femur 416
- Knee region 417
  - Knee joint movement 417
  - Ageing related knee injuries 419
  - Sports related knee injuries 420
  - Common Fibular Nerve Injury 421
  - Knee joint injury 423

Lachman's Test 425

Ankle Region 425

    Ankle injury associated with sports 427

    Ankle injuries associated with ageing 428

    Ankle joint dysfunction 429

    Pott's Fracture 431

    Sprained Ankle 432

Chapter 11: Vertebral Column Injury 433

Introduction 433

    Motor symptoms caused by vertebral column injury 434

    Treatment of vertebral column injury 436

Cervical vertebrae 439

    Cervical vertebral injury 439

Lumbar vertebrae 440

    Lumbar Injury 440

    Lower back pain 443

    Herniation of nucleus pulposus 444

Chapter 12: Methods for diagnosing and assessing motor dysfunction 446

Methods 446

Examples 448

Neuroimaging 449

    Common types of neuroimaging 450

    Application of neuroimaging 451

    Neuroimaging and Pakinson's disease 452

    Neuroimaging and multiple sclerosis 455

    Neuroimaging and stroke 457

    Neuroimaging and spinal cord injury 458

Chapter 13: Future directions in motor control research 463

References 465

Index 468

CHAPTER 1: INTRODUCTION TO MOVEMENT CONTROL

Movement control refers to the complex process by which the human body produces, coordinates, and regulates movement. Movement control is essential for everyday activities such as walking, reaching, and grasping, as well as more complex activities such as sports, dance, and music.

The nervous system plays a central role in movement control. The brain, spinal cord, and peripheral nerves work together to initiate and coordinate movements. The brain plays a critical role in planning and controlling movement, while the spinal cord and peripheral nerves execute the movement.

There are several key structures and systems involved in movement control, including:

1. Motor cortex: The motor cortex is a region of the brain responsible for planning, initiating, and executing movement.

The motor cortex is divided into different regions, each responsible for controlling specific movements.

2. Basal ganglia: The basal ganglia are a group of nuclei located deep within the brain. The basal ganglia are involved in the regulation of voluntary movements and play a critical role in the initiation and termination of movements.

3. Cerebellum: The cerebellum is a region of the brain located at the base of the skull. The cerebellum is involved in the coordination and regulation of movement, including the maintenance of balance and posture.

4. Spinal cord: The spinal cord is a long, thin bundle of nerves that extends from the brain down through the back. The spinal cord is responsible for relaying information between the brain and the rest of the body and plays a critical role in the execution of movement.

5. Muscles: Muscles are the key structures responsible for generating force and producing movement. The contraction of muscles is controlled by the nervous system, and muscles work together in a coordinated manner to produce smooth and efficient movement.

6. Sensory systems: Sensory systems provide feedback to the nervous system during movement, allowing for the continuous modification and adjustment of movement. The somatosensory system provides information about the position and movement

of the body, while the visual and vestibular systems provide information about the environment and movement in relation to the environment.

Therefore, movement control is a complex process that involves the interaction of multiple structures and systems within the body. The nervous system plays a central role in movement control, while the key structures and systems involved in movement include the motor cortex, basal ganglia, cerebellum, spinal cord, muscles, and sensory systems. Understanding the principles of movement control is essential for the development of effective interventions for movement disorders and for the improvement of human movement performance in a variety of contexts.

HUMAN BRAIN

Broadmann's Brain Map

Brodmann's human brain map, also known as Brodmann's areas, is a map of the human brain based on the organization of its cellular structure (Fig. 1.1). It was created by German neurologist and psychiatrist Korbinian Brodmann in the early 20th century.

Brodmann divided the cortex into 52 distinct areas based on differences in the size, shape, and organization of neurons in each region. He used a staining technique called the Nissl stain to identify these differences in the cellular structure.

Each Brodmann area is numbered and corresponds to a specific region of the brain that is thought to have a unique function. For example, Brodmann area 17, located in the occipital lobe, is responsible for processing visual information, while Brodmann area 44 and 45, located in the frontal lobe, are involved in language production and comprehension.

Brodmann's areas have been widely used by neuroscientists to study the structure and function of the human brain. They provide a common framework for describing brain regions across different studies and have helped researchers to identify specific regions of interest for various neurological and psychiatric conditions.

However, it is important to note that the function of each Brodmann area is not completely understood and may vary across individuals. Modern neuroimaging techniques, such as functional magnetic resonance imaging (fMRI), have provided further insight into the functional organization of the brain.

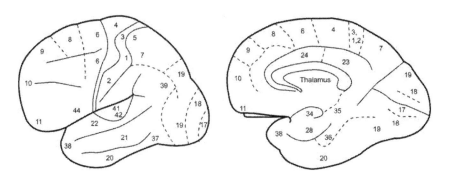

Chapter 1: Introduction to movement control

Figure 1. Brodmann's map

Figure 1.1. Brodmann's human brain map. The top is the lateral view, and the bottom is the medial view. The numbers are Brodman's brain areas.

Primary Motor Map

The primary motor map, also known as the motor homunculus, is a representation of the body's muscles and their corresponding motor neurons in the brain's primary motor cortex. It is a topographic map, meaning that adjacent areas of the body are represented in adjacent areas of the cortex.

The primary motor cortex lies anterior to the central sulcus (Brodmann's area 4 or M1). The functional complexity of movements determines the size of the primary motor cortical area, such that the fingers and face require a large area of the somatomotor cortex (Fig. 1.1). In contrast, a much smaller area is devoted to the body, trunk, and proximal limbs because they only need gross motor activity.

The size of each body part's representation on the motor map is proportional to the complexity of its movement. For example, the hands and face occupy a disproportionately large area of the motor map compared to their size in the body, reflecting the intricate movements they are capable of.

The motor map is crucial for the planning and execution of voluntary movements, as it provides a spatial organization of motor commands that are sent to the muscles. Dysfunction or damage to the motor cortex can result in motor deficits or paralysis of the corresponding body parts.

The following sections describe the relationship between the areas of M1 and the skeletal muscles. They also describe the functional aspects of a single pyramidal tract neuron in presetting, force, precision, and orientation of voluntary movement control.

The primary motor map indicates the cortical area controlling motor function. It shows the relationship between the cortical areas and muscle groups. The pattern of organization is such that the top part of the primary motor cortex controls the lower part of the body. In comparison, the lower part of the primary motor cortex controls the upper part of the body. Therefore, the pattern of the primary motor map in regulating body parts is in reverse order.

Another important feature is that the size of the representative area of the primary motor cortex depends on the preciseness and complexity required for the movement. For example, the finger takes up a much greater area of the primary motor cortex than the toe. The thigh has a small area supplied by the primary motor cortex compared with the size of the cortical area supplying the hand in relative proportion.

Chapter 1: Introduction to movement control

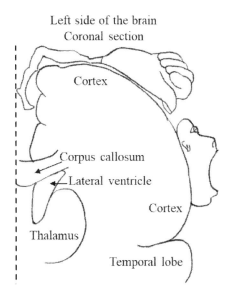

Figure 2

Figure 1.2. Functional representation of the primary motor cortex. The images are superimposed on a coronal plane of the brain, which shows that the more complex the movement, the larger the cortical representation area. There is a reverse order: the lower end of the precentral gyrus represents the face. The paracentral lobule on the medial surface of the cerebral hemisphere represents the leg. Damage to cortical motor neurons causes little or no atrophy in muscles. Abbreviations: cc: corpus callosum; LV: lateral ventricle; Tha: thalamus.

Cortical Columns

Cortical columns are formed by a group of neurons accumulating together in the cortex, arranged in a vertical unit. The neurons within a cortical column usually share a similar morphology and function. These neurons commonly work together for particular functions. The neurons within a cortical column usually share common input and output connections. A cortical column is a basic unit for cortical information processing.

Cortical lamina organization

The lamina organization of the human cortex consists of six layers. These six layers, from the brain surface downward, are the molecular, external granular, external pyramidal, internal granular, internal pyramidal, and multiform layers. The molecular layer (layer I) mainly consists of axons and dendrites with very few cell bodies. The external granular layer (layer II) contains densely packed small cells, including pyramidal and stellate cells. The external pyramidal layer (layer III) features medium-sized pyramidal cells. The internal granular layer (layer IV) contains densely packed stellate and pyramidal cells. The internal pyramidal layer (layer V) consists of large to medium-sized pyramidal cells. Finally, the multiform layer (layer VI) features irregularly shaped cells.

Chapter 1: Introduction to movement control

Cellular layers of the somatomotor cortex

The somatomotor cortex is organized into six layers. However, the differences between the primary and association motor cortex are seen in the cytoarchitecture. The primary motor cortex has the largest neurons, called *Betz cells*, in layer V of the primary motor cortex. The largest Betz cells are in the upper part of the primary motor cortex, whereas the neurons supply the muscles of the lower limbs. Therefore, the size of the neurons, such as Betz cells, is related to the size of the muscles. This is the morphology of a neuron, which, in many aspects, reflects the function. Similarly, this concept is also reflected in layer IV of the somatomotor cortex. Layer IV is the internal granular layer consisting of densely packed and small-sized granular cells. However, layer IV of the somatomotor cortex is very thin and contains virtually no internal granular cell layer. The somatomotor cortex is also called the *agranular cortex.*

Damage to the cortical motor neurons causes little or no atrophy in the muscle. This is because only lower motor neurons supply nutritional nerve factors to the muscle, not the upper motor neurons.

Cortical homunculus

Homunculus is a Latin word meaning "little man." Here, the cortex means the primary and association motor cortices. A *cortical homunculus* (Fig. 1.2 below) is a representation of the human body based on a neurological map of the areas and proportions of the human brain regulating movements for different parts of the body.

The cortical homunculus is a representation of the human body in the somatosensory cortex, which is the part of the brain that processes information related to touch, pain, temperature, and proprioception (the sense of where the body is in space). The homunculus is a distorted, caricature-like map of the body, where the size of each body part is proportional to the amount of cortical area dedicated to processing sensory information from that body part.

The cortical homunculus was first described by the Canadian neurosurgeon Wilder Penfield in the 1930s, who mapped the somatosensory cortex by electrically stimulating different areas of the brain in awake patients undergoing brain surgery. His findings revealed that specific areas of the cortex were responsible for processing information from different parts of the body, and that these areas were arranged in a somatotopic manner, with adjacent areas corresponding to adjacent parts of the body.

Chapter 1: Introduction to movement control

The homunculus is often depicted as a distorted figure, with the face, hands, and lips disproportionately large, reflecting the high degree of sensory processing devoted to these areas. In contrast, the torso and legs are relatively small in the homunculus, reflecting the smaller amount of cortical area dedicated to processing sensory information from these body parts.

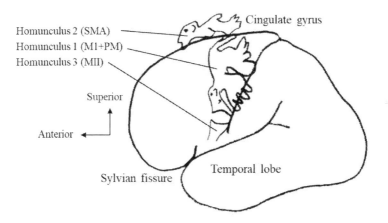

Figure 1.3. Homunculi 1, 2 and 3

Homunculus 1 is composed of Brodmann's areas 4 (M1) and 6 (PM). Control of muscles by the cortex is largely contralateral (opposite side). For example, the left primary motor cortex controls the muscles on the right side of the body. Some muscles are bilaterally controlled, such as those in the upper part of the face, those used for mastication, and those in the soft palate, larynx, and trunk.

The somatomotor neurons lie in layer 5 of the somatomotor cortex and are somatotopically organized. In homunculus 1, the neurons supplying the facial muscles are in the lower end. The neurons supplying the arm and hand muscles are higher in the upper part of homunculus 1. The neurons supplying the proximal part of the body are in the rostral part of homunculus 1.

Homunculus 2 lies in the superior medial part of area 6, or the *supplementary motor area*. It has the following features:

The threshold to elicit movement needs to be higher in homunculus 2 than in homunculus 1. The precision of somatotopic representation is poor in homunculus 2. Activation of muscles by homunculus 2 is extensive and typically extends to more than one joint. Homunculus 2 contributes primarily to bilateral movements for maintaining posture.

Homunculus 3 lies in the most inferolateral part of the precentral gyrus and extends into the Sylvian fissure. The functional organization of homunculus 3 is not clear.

Chapter 1: Introduction to movement control

Somatosensory cortex

Sensory information inputs influence motor control. Sensory information inputs are derived from peripheral stimulations, such as light, temperature, and sound. The sensors located inside the target organ receive a signal of peripheral stimulation. The information is then sent to the brain, which, in turn, can influence motor function.

The *somatosensory cortex* senses the information derived from the peripheral target organs. It lies behind the central sulcus and can be divided into three major categories according to their respective functions related to motor control (Fig. 1.4).

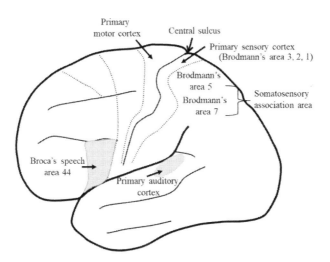

Figure 1.4. Somatosensory cortex

- The first part is called the *primary sensory cortex* and is mainly used for sensing information inputs. The primary sensory area is found behind the central sulcus and is parallel to the primary motor cortex, which is in front of the central sulcus. The primary sensory cortex is equivalent to Brodmann's areas 3, 1, and 2, from upper to lower positions.

- The second part is called the *somatosensory association area*, which is related to the integration and classification of types of information inputs. The somatosensory association area lies posterior to the primary sensory cortex. The somatosensory association cortex is equivalent to Brodmann's areas 5 and 7 and lies posterior to the primary sensory cortex. Brodmann's area 5 lies above Brodmann's area 7. The functions of the two are different and will be detailed in the latter part of this book.
- The third part is related to specific inputs from the primary visual field and primary auditory area. The primary visual field can be found along the calcarine sulcus in the occipital lobe. The primary auditory cortex lies just below the lateral fissure in the superior temporal lobe. Broca's speech area 44 is also a somatosensory association cortex and lies anterior to the inferior part of the premotor cortex.

Sensory input

Sensory input to the somatomotor cortex originates from skin, muscles, and joints. Skin, muscles, and joints have sensory apparatus, which can generate signals in response to stimulation. The information is first sent to the spinal cord and then to the thalamus. After changing neurons in the thalamus, the information is sent to the primary sensory cortex. In general, there is very little direct input from the peripheral organ to the primary sensory cortex.

Cortical-cortical connections

The control of movement is a complex process that involves multiple regions of the brain, including the cortex and its connections. Here are some key cortical regions and connections involved in motor control:

1. Primary motor cortex: Located in the frontal lobe, this area is responsible for the execution of voluntary movements. It sends signals to the muscles of the body via descending motor pathways, such as the corticospinal tract.
2. Premotor cortex: Located in the frontal lobe, this area is involved in the planning and preparation of movements. It receives input from various sensory and motor areas of the brain and helps to coordinate complex movements.
3. Supplementary motor area: Located in the medial frontal lobe, this area is involved in the initiation and coordination of movements, particularly those involving both hands.
4. Posterior parietal cortex: Located in the parietal lobe, this area is involved in integrating sensory information from multiple modalities to guide movements. It plays a key role in spatial

awareness and in generating motor plans that are adapted to the environment.

5. Basal ganglia: This group of subcortical structures is involved in the selection and initiation of movements, as well as in learning and habit formation. It receives input from the cortex and sends signals back to the cortex via thalamocortical pathways.
6. Cerebellum: This structure is involved in the coordination and refinement of movements, as well as in motor learning and error correction. It receives input from the cortex and sends signals back via the thalamus.
7. Thalamus: This subcortical structure acts as a relay station between the cortex and other parts of the brain, including the basal ganglia and cerebellum. It is involved in the processing and integration of sensory information related to movement.

These cortical regions and connections work together to plan, execute, and refine movements with precision and accuracy. Dysfunction or damage to any of these areas can result in motor deficits or impairments in motor control.

The pathway of the motor control system consists of three major parts. These are: (1) sensory input from the peripheral nervous system, (2) information processing within the brain, and (3) motor output projecting to the lower motor neurons in the spinal cord.

Chapter 1: Introduction to movement control

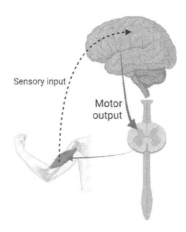

Figure 1.5. An example of motor control pathway

MOTOR CONTROL THEORIES

There are several theories of motor control, each of which provides a unique perspective on how the brain controls and coordinates movement. Three of the most prominent theories are the hierarchical model, the systems model, and the ecological model. Let's take a closer look at each of these theories.

Hierarchical, system, and ecological models

Hierarchical Model: The hierarchical model is a top-down approach to motor control that suggests that the brain controls movement through a series of levels, with each level being responsible for a different aspect of movement control. The levels include the highest level of the cortex, down to the spinal cord and peripheral nerves. The higher levels of the brain plan and initiate movement, while lower levels are responsible for executing the movements. This model suggests that each level of the system works together to create smooth and coordinated movement. However, some criticisms of this model suggest that it oversimplifies the complexity of motor control and does not account for the many feedback loops that occur during movement.

Systems Model: The systems model proposes that motor control arises from the interaction of many different subsystems, each contributing to the overall control of movement. This model suggests that there is no single "control center" for movement, but rather that movement is controlled by the interaction of many different subsystems, including sensory systems, musculoskeletal systems, and neural systems. This model emphasizes the importance of feedback in motor control, suggesting that movements are constantly modified and adjusted based on sensory input.

Ecological Model: The ecological model emphasizes the importance of the environment in shaping movement control. This model suggests that the perception of the environment is just as important as the perception of the body in controlling movement. In this model, movement is seen as emerging from the interaction between the body and the environment, rather than being controlled solely by the brain. This model also emphasizes the importance of context in shaping movement, suggesting that

Chapter 1: Introduction to movement control

movement is influenced by factors such as social and cultural norms, as well as individual goals and intentions.

In summary, each of these models offers a unique perspective on motor control. The hierarchical model emphasizes the importance of top-down control from the brain, the systems model highlights the importance of the interaction between multiple subsystems, and the ecological model emphasizes the importance of the environment and context in shaping movement control.

Here are some examples of each of the motor control models:

Hierarchical Model: The hierarchical model can be seen in the control of voluntary movements. For example, when you decide to lift your arm to reach for a cup, the highest level of the brain's motor cortex initiates the movement, while lower levels of the brain, the spinal cord, and the peripheral nerves execute the movement. This model also applies to the control of more complex movements, such as walking, where the brain plans and initiates the movement, and the lower levels of the nervous system, including the spinal cord and muscles, execute the movement.

Systems Model: The systems model can be seen in the control of balance during movement. For example, when walking on an uneven surface, such as a rocky trail, your balance control system integrates sensory information from your vision, inner ear, and somatosensory system to continuously adjust and modulate muscle activity to maintain balance. This model also applies to the control of more complex movements, such as throwing a ball, where the subsystems of vision, proprioception, and motor control all work together to adjust the movement based on feedback.

Ecological Model: The ecological model can be seen in the control of movement in everyday life. For example, when reaching for an object on a cluttered desk, your movement control is influenced by the layout of the environment and the location of the object. This model also applies to the control of more complex movements, such as playing a team sport like basketball, where movement is shaped by social and cultural norms, such as the rules of the game and the strategies employed by the team.

Somatic motor control hierarchy

Somatic motor control refers to the regulation of voluntary movement of skeletal muscles, which is controlled by a hierarchical system in the brain. The somatic motor control hierarchy can be divided into three main levels:

1. Spinal Level: The spinal cord is the lowest level of the hierarchy, and it is responsible for generating basic reflexive movements, such as the withdrawal reflex. Reflexes are rapid, automatic, and stereotyped responses to sensory input that do not require conscious thought or control.

Chapter 1: Introduction to movement control

2. Brainstem Level: The brainstem is the intermediate level of the hierarchy and includes several important structures, such as the medulla, pons, and midbrain. These structures are involved in regulating posture and balance, as well as in controlling eye movements, facial expressions, and chewing and swallowing. The brainstem also contains nuclei that are important for controlling respiration and cardiovascular function, which are essential for supporting movement.
3. Cerebral Level: The cerebral cortex is the highest level of the hierarchy and is responsible for the planning, execution, and control of voluntary movements. The cerebral cortex can be further divided into the following regions:
4. Primary Motor Cortex: Located in the precentral gyrus of the frontal lobe, this region is responsible for generating motor commands that control voluntary movements. It receives input from other areas of the cortex, including the premotor cortex and posterior parietal cortex, as well as from subcortical structures such as the basal ganglia and cerebellum.
5. Premotor Cortex: Located in the frontal lobe, this region is involved in the planning and preparation of movements. It receives input from sensory areas of the cortex and integrates this information to generate motor plans.
6. Posterior Parietal Cortex: Located in the parietal lobe, this region is involved in integrating sensory information from multiple modalities to guide movements. It plays a key role in

spatial awareness and in generating motor plans that are adapted to the environment.
7. Basal Ganglia and Cerebellum: These subcortical structures are involved in the selection and refinement of movements. They receive input from the cortex and provide feedback to the cortex via thalamocortical pathways.

The somatic motor control hierarchy is organized in a hierarchical manner, with each level contributing to the generation and control of voluntary movement. Dysfunction or damage to any level of the hierarchy can result in motor deficits or impairments in motor control.

Chapter 1: Introduction to movement control

The table summarises the somatomotor control hierarchy

Level of Control	Brain Region	Function
Spinal Level	Spinal Cord	Generates basic reflexive movements
Brainstem Level	Medulla, Pons, Midbrain	Regulates posture, balance, eye movements, facial expressions, chewing and swallowing, respiration, and cardiovascular function
Cerebral Level	Cerebral Cortex	Plans, executes, and controls voluntary movements
- Primary Motor Cortex	Precentral Gyrus of the Frontal Lobe	Generates motor commands that control voluntary movements
- Premotor Cortex	Frontal Lobe	Involved in the planning and preparation of movements
- Posterior Parietal Cortex	Parietal Lobe	Integrates sensory information to guide movements
- Basal Ganglia	Subcortical Structures	Selects and refines movements
- Cerebellum	Subcortical Structures	Coordinates and refines movements, and plays a role in motor learning and error correction

SENSORIMOTOR INTEGRATION

Sensorimotor integration is the process by which the sensory and motor systems work together to control movement. It involves the integration of sensory information from various sources, such as vision, touch, and proprioception, to guide motor output and produce appropriate movements.

Sensory information is processed and integrated at various levels of the nervous system, from the peripheral sensory receptors to the central nervous system. The sensory information is then used to generate appropriate motor commands, which are sent to the muscles to produce movement.

The sensory information is processed in a hierarchical manner, with lower-level sensory information being integrated at the spinal cord level and higher-level sensory information being processed in the brain. For example, when a person touches a hot surface, the sensory information from the skin is processed at the spinal cord level, which triggers a reflex response to withdraw the hand. This reflex response is an example of a lower-level sensory-motor integration.

In contrast, higher-level sensory-motor integration involves the integration of sensory information from multiple sources and the processing of this information in the brain. For example, when a person reaches for an object, the brain integrates visual, proprioceptive, and tactile information to generate the appropriate motor commands to reach and grasp the object.

The cerebellum, which is located at the base of the brain, plays a crucial role in sensorimotor integration. It receives input from the sensory and motor systems and is involved in the coordination and timing of movements. The cerebellum helps to ensure that movements are smooth and accurate by constantly monitoring and adjusting the motor commands based on the sensory feedback received during movement.

Chapter 1: Introduction to movement control

In summary, sensorimotor integration is a complex process that involves the integration of sensory information from multiple sources to generate appropriate motor commands. This process is essential for the production of smooth and accurate movements and is facilitated by the cerebellum and other structures within the nervous system.

Here are a few examples of how the sensory and motor systems work together to control movement through sensorimotor integration:

1. Reaching and grasping: When reaching for an object, the brain integrates sensory information from vision, proprioception (sense of limb position), and touch to generate the appropriate motor commands to reach and grasp the object. This involves the coordination of multiple muscles in the arm and hand to produce a smooth and accurate movement.

2. Walking on an uneven surface: When walking on an uneven surface, the sensory information from the feet and legs is processed in the spinal cord and brain to generate the appropriate motor commands to adjust the muscles in the legs and maintain balance. The cerebellum plays a crucial role in this process by constantly monitoring and adjusting the motor commands based on the sensory feedback received during movement.

3. Catching a ball: When catching a ball, the brain integrates visual information about the trajectory of the ball and proprioceptive information from the hands and arms to generate the appropriate motor commands to position the hands and fingers to catch the ball. This involves the coordination of multiple muscles in the hands and arms to produce a smooth and accurate movement.

4. Typing on a keyboard: When typing on a keyboard, the brain integrates visual information about the location of the keys and proprioceptive information from the fingers and hands to generate the appropriate motor commands to press the keys. This involves the coordination of multiple muscles in the fingers and hands to produce a smooth and accurate movement.

In each of these cases, sensorimotor integration is essential for producing smooth and accurate movements, and involves the integration of sensory information from multiple sources to generate appropriate motor commands.

Therefore, the sensory and motor systems work together to control movement, including that sensory information is processed and integrated to guide motor output.

CHAPTER 2: MOTOR LEARNING

Motor learning is the process of acquiring and improving motor skills through practice and experience. Motor skills are abilities that enable individuals to perform movements and actions, such as walking, running, throwing, and typing. The development of motor skills occurs throughout the lifespan, starting from infancy and continuing into adulthood.

The acquisition and improvement of motor skills involve multiple stages, including the cognitive stage, the associative stage, and the autonomous stage. During the cognitive stage, individuals are focused on understanding the task and developing a basic understanding of the movement. In the associative stage, individuals refine their movements and develop a more consistent technique. In the autonomous stage, movements become automatic and require less conscious effort to perform.

Feedback, practice, and environmental factors all play a role in motor learning. Feedback provides information about the quality and accuracy of motor performance and can be intrinsic or extrinsic.

Practice is necessary for motor skill acquisition and improvement, and the type and frequency of practice can impact motor learning outcomes. Environmental factors such as equipment, coaching, and social support can also influence motor skill development.

Motor learning principles are applied in various settings, including sports, physical therapy, and occupational therapy. Understanding the principles of motor learning can help individuals and professionals enhance motor skill performance and improve quality of life.

INTRODUCTION TO MOTOR LEARNING

Basic concept of motor learning

The basic concept of motor learning is the acquisition and improvement of motor skills through practice and experience. Motor skills are abilities that enable individuals to perform movements and actions, such as walking, running, throwing, and typing. Motor learning is a complex process that involves multiple stages, including the cognitive stage, the associative stage, and the autonomous stage. Feedback, practice, and environmental factors all play a role in motor learning. Feedback provides information about the quality and accuracy of motor performance and can be intrinsic or extrinsic. Practice is necessary for motor skill acquisition and improvement, and the type and frequency of practice can impact motor learning outcomes. Environmental factors such as equipment, coaching, and social support can also influence motor skill development.

Motor learning principles are applied in various settings, including sports, physical therapy, and occupational therapy. Understanding the principles of motor learning can help individuals and professionals enhance motor skill performance and improve quality of life.

Types of motor skills

There are several types of motor skills that are relevant to motor learning. Here are some of the main types:

1. Gross motor skills: These involve large muscle groups and typically relate to activities like running, jumping, and throwing.
2. Fine motor skills: These involve small muscle groups and typically relate to activities like writing, typing, and playing musical instruments.
3. Discrete motor skills: These involve specific, well-defined movements that have a clear beginning and end. Examples include hitting a baseball or throwing a dart.
4. Continuous motor skills: These involve movements that have no clear beginning or end and are performed for an extended period of time. Examples include walking, running, and swimming.

5. Serial motor skills: These involve a sequence of discrete movements performed in a particular order. Examples include playing a musical instrument or typing on a keyboard.

6. Closed motor skills: These are performed in a predictable and stable environment, where the performer has control over the timing and execution of the movement. Examples include hitting a golf ball or shooting a free throw in basketball.

7. Open motor skills: These are performed in an unpredictable and constantly changing environment, where the performer must adapt their movement to external factors. Examples include playing a team sport or driving a car in traffic.

Understanding the different types of motor skills is important for designing effective motor learning programs and interventions. Different types of motor skills may require different practice schedules, feedback strategies, and environmental conditions to optimize skill acquisition and performance.

Stages of motor learning

There are three main stages of motor learning that individuals typically progress through as they acquire and refine motor skills. These stages are:

1. Cognitive stage: In the cognitive stage, learners are focused on understanding the task and developing a basic understanding of the movement. During this stage, learners may rely on verbal

instructions, demonstrations, and visual aids to help them understand how to perform the movement. They may also make frequent errors and require a lot of feedback to improve their performance.

2. Associative stage: In the associative stage, learners begin to refine their movements and develop a more consistent technique. During this stage, learners become more self-aware and able to detect errors on their own. They may also begin to incorporate more subtle movements and adjust their technique based on feedback. The goal of this stage is to reduce variability and increase the accuracy and efficiency of the movement.

3. Autonomous stage: In the autonomous stage, movements become automatic and require less conscious effort to perform. During this stage, learners are able to perform the movement with minimal errors and without much attention. They may also be able to adapt their technique to different environments and situations. The goal of this stage is to develop a high level of skill and efficiency in the movement.

Understanding the different stages of motor learning is important for designing effective learning and practice strategies. Learners in different stages may require different types and amounts of feedback, practice schedules, and environmental conditions to optimize their performance and progress to the next stage of learning.

Motor skill acquisition and retention

There are several factors that can influence motor skill acquisition and retention. Here are some of the most important ones:

1. Practice: Practice is the most important factor that influences motor skill acquisition and retention. The amount and quality of practice can significantly affect how quickly and effectively learners acquire and retain motor skills.

2. Feedback: Feedback is also critical for motor skill acquisition and retention. Feedback provides learners with information about the quality and accuracy of their performance, and allows them to make adjustments to their movements to improve their skill.

3. Environmental factors: Environmental factors, such as the type of equipment, coaching, and social support, can also influence motor skill acquisition and retention. For example, having access to high-quality equipment or working with a skilled coach can enhance learning and retention.

4. Individual factors: Individual factors, such as age, gender, and physical ability, can also affect motor skill acquisition and retention. For example, younger learners may acquire motor skills more quickly than older learners, and males may have an advantage in some types of motor skills compared to females.

5. Cognitive processes: Cognitive processes, such as attention, memory, and problem-solving, are also important for motor

skill acquisition and retention. Learners who are able to pay close attention to their movements, remember the steps involved, and solve problems that arise during practice are more likely to acquire and retain motor skills.

6. Transfer of learning: The ability to transfer motor skills learned in one context to another context is also important for motor skill acquisition and retention. Learners who are able to apply their skills to new situations and environments are more likely to retain those skills over time.

Understanding these factors can help instructors and coaches design effective motor learning programs and interventions that optimize skill acquisition and retention.

FEEDBACK

Feedback in motor learning

Feedback is critical for motor learning as it provides learners with information about the quality and accuracy of their movements. Feedback can come in various forms, such as verbal instructions, demonstrations, and visual aids, and it can be provided by instructors, coaches, or technology.

Here are some of the main reasons why feedback is important for motor learning:

1. Error detection and correction: Feedback allows learners to identify errors in their movements and make corrections to improve their technique. Without feedback, learners may continue to make the same mistakes, which can hinder their skill acquisition and performance.

2. Reinforcement of correct movements: Feedback can reinforce correct movements by providing learners with positive reinforcement when they perform a movement correctly. This positive reinforcement can increase the likelihood that the learner will repeat the correct movement in the future.

3. Motivation: Feedback can also be motivational for learners, as it provides them with a sense of progress and accomplishment. Learners who receive positive feedback are more likely to feel motivated to continue practicing and improving their skills.

4. Informational value: Feedback provides learners with information about the movement, such as its timing, trajectory, and force. This information can help learners develop a better understanding of the movement and how to execute it more effectively.

5. Generalization of skills: Feedback can also help learners generalize their skills to new contexts and environments. By providing feedback that highlights the key elements of the movement, learners can develop a deeper understanding of the underlying principles of the movement, which can help them apply the skill in new situations.

Chapter 2: Motor learning

Overall, feedback is a critical component of motor learning as it provides learners with information about their movements and helps them develop a better understanding of the skill. By providing effective feedback, instructors and coaches can help learners acquire and retain motor skills more effectively.

Feedback be used to improve motor skills

Feedback can be used in various ways to improve motor skills. Here are some strategies that instructors and coaches can use to effectively utilize feedback to improve motor skills:

1. Provide immediate feedback: Immediate feedback can be more effective in helping learners improve their motor skills compared to delayed feedback. Instructors and coaches should aim to provide feedback as soon as possible after the movement is performed to help learners make adjustments in real-time.

2. Focus on specific aspects of the movement: Feedback should be focused on specific aspects of the movement that need improvement. By identifying the specific areas that require improvement, learners can focus their efforts on making targeted improvements to their technique.

3. Use different types of feedback: Feedback can come in various forms, such as verbal instructions, demonstrations, and visual aids. Instructors and coaches should use a combination of

feedback types to help learners develop a comprehensive understanding of the movement.

4. Gradually reduce feedback: As learners improve their motor skills, instructors and coaches should gradually reduce the amount of feedback provided. This can help learners develop greater self-awareness and rely less on external feedback over time.

5. Encourage self-reflection: Instructors and coaches should encourage learners to reflect on their own performance and provide their own feedback. This can help learners develop a greater sense of self-awareness and take ownership of their own learning and development.

By effectively utilizing feedback, instructors and coaches can help learners improve their motor skills more quickly and effectively. Providing timely and targeted feedback, using a variety of feedback types, and encouraging self-reflection can all contribute to effective feedback strategies for motor skill acquisition and improvement.

Intrinsic feedback of motor learning

Intrinsic feedback refers to the sensory information that the learner receives from their own body during the execution of a movement or skill. This feedback comes from the proprioceptive, vestibular, and visual systems, which provide information about the position, movement, and orientation of the body.

Chapter 2: Motor learning

For example, when a learner performs a golf swing, they receive intrinsic feedback from their own body through the sensory information provided by their muscles and joints. This feedback allows them to adjust their movements in real-time to improve their technique.

Intrinsic feedback is an important component of motor learning as it provides learners with immediate information about their movements. However, it is important to note that intrinsic feedback is not always accurate or reliable. Factors such as fatigue, pain, and injury can all affect the sensory information received by the learner, which can in turn affect their ability to learn and perform motor skills.

Therefore, instructors and coaches often supplement intrinsic feedback with extrinsic feedback, which is feedback provided by an external source such as a coach or technology. By using a combination of intrinsic and extrinsic feedback, learners can develop a more complete understanding of their movements and improve their motor skills more effectively.

Example:

When a learner performs a tennis serve, they receive intrinsic feedback from their own body through the sensory information provided by their muscles and joints. For example, the learner may feel the stretch in their shoulder and arm as they begin the windup phase of the serve. As they initiate the throwing motion, they may feel the tension in their wrist and fingers as they grip the racket. During the follow-through phase, they may feel the contraction in their abdominal muscles as they rotate their torso to generate power.

This intrinsic feedback can help the learner adjust their movements in real-time to improve their technique. For example, if the learner notices that they are not generating enough power in their serve, they may adjust their follow-through to increase the rotation of their torso, which would result in a more powerful serve.

However, it is important to note that intrinsic feedback is not always reliable or accurate. For example, if the learner is fatigued or has an injury, the sensory information they receive from their own body may be distorted or misleading. In such cases, extrinsic feedback from a coach or technology may be necessary to supplement and validate the intrinsic feedback.

Extrinsic feedback of motor learning

Extrinsic feedback is feedback that is provided by an external source, such as a coach, technology, or another person. It is used to supplement and enhance the intrinsic feedback that a learner receives from their own body during the execution of a movement or skill.

Extrinsic feedback can be either knowledge of results (KR), which is feedback about the outcome or result of a movement, or knowledge of performance (KP), which is feedback about the quality of the movement itself.

For example, if a learner is practicing a golf swing, a coach may provide extrinsic feedback in the form of KR by telling the learner how far the ball traveled or KP by pointing out a flaw in their technique, such as an incorrect grip or a misaligned posture.

Extrinsic feedback can be provided in various forms, such as verbal instructions, demonstrations, or visual aids. It can be used to reinforce correct movements, correct errors, and provide motivation and encouragement to learners.

Extrinsic feedback is an important component of motor learning, as it can help learners develop a more complete understanding of their movements and improve their technique more effectively. However, it is important to note that extrinsic feedback should be used in conjunction with intrinsic feedback, as over-reliance on extrinsic feedback can hinder the development of a learner's self-awareness and self-correction skills.

PRACTICE

The role of practice

Practice is a critical component of motor learning, as it allows learners to repeatedly perform and refine their movements to improve their skill level. Through practice, learners can develop the necessary neural pathways and muscle memory to execute movements more efficiently and effectively.

There are different types of practice schedules that can be used to enhance motor learning, including:

1. Massed practice: This involves performing a large amount of practice in a short amount of time, with minimal rest breaks in between. Massed practice can be useful for developing endurance and for improving performance in simple, well-learned tasks.

2. Distributed practice: This involves breaking up practice sessions into shorter, more frequent sessions with rest intervals in between. Distributed practice can be more effective for learning complex skills and for retaining information over longer periods of time.

3. Blocked practice: This involves practicing the same skill or movement repeatedly in a blocked or consistent manner. Blocked practice can be useful for beginners to develop the fundamental movements and can provide a sense of consistency and control.

4. Random practice: This involves practicing multiple skills or movements in a random or variable order. Random practice can be more effective for developing transferable skills and for improving retention and long-term learning.

The type of practice schedule used depends on the skill level of the learner, the nature of the task, and the goals of the practice. In general, a combination of different practice schedules can be used to enhance motor learning and facilitate skill acquisition.

Practice impact skill acquisition and retention

Practice is a critical factor in motor skill acquisition and retention. Regular and consistent practice is necessary for learners to develop the necessary neural pathways and muscle memory to execute movements more efficiently and effectively.

During practice, learners go through the stages of motor learning, which includes the cognitive stage, the associative stage, and the autonomous stage. As learners progress through these stages, their movements become more automatic, efficient, and consistent.

In addition to improving skill acquisition, practice can also enhance the retention of motor skills. When learners practice a skill repeatedly over time, they are more likely to retain the information and be able to execute the skill accurately and consistently over longer periods.

However, the type of practice used can impact the effectiveness of motor skill acquisition and retention.

- Research has shown that distributed practice, where practice sessions are broken up into shorter, more frequent sessions

with rest intervals in between, can be more effective for retaining motor skills over longer periods.
- In contrast, massed practice, where a large amount of practice is performed in a short amount of time, can be effective for developing endurance and improving performance in simple, well-learned tasks, but may not be as effective for long-term retention.

The use of feedback during practice can also impact motor skill acquisition and retention. Feedback can help learners adjust their movements in real-time, correct errors, and reinforce correct movements. Providing feedback at appropriate intervals during practice can enhance learning and retention of motor skills.

Overall, consistent and well-designed practice, with appropriate feedback and rest intervals, is essential for motor skill acquisition and retention.

What is the deliberate practice?

Deliberate practice is a type of practice that is designed to improve performance and enhance learning in a specific skill or domain. It involves engaging in highly structured and focused practice sessions that are specifically designed to challenge the learner and push them beyond their current skill level.

Deliberate practice typically involves breaking down a skill into smaller components and practicing each component in isolation

Chapter 2: Motor learning

before integrating them back into the whole skill. It also involves setting specific goals, receiving immediate feedback, and adjusting practice based on that feedback.

Deliberate practice is often used in sports, music, and other performance-based domains, where high levels of skill are required. However, it can also be applied to other areas such as academic subjects, language learning, and even everyday tasks.

Research has shown that deliberate practice can significantly improve skill acquisition and performance. It can also enhance motivation and self-efficacy, as learners see progress and improvements in their skills through focused and intentional practice. However, deliberate practice can be demanding and requires significant effort and persistence, making it more challenging for some learners to engage in than others.

Let's say you want to improve your ability to play the piano. Instead of simply playing through your favorite songs or practicing random exercises, you engage in deliberate practice. This involves breaking down the skill of playing the piano into smaller components, such as hand placement, finger dexterity, and sight-reading.

You then set specific goals for each component, such as being able to play a specific chord progression smoothly, or sight-reading a specific piece of music at a certain tempo. You then engage in focused and intentional practice sessions, focusing on each component one at a time, and adjusting your practice based on immediate feedback. For example, you might record yourself playing and then analyze the recording to identify areas where you can improve your technique or timing.

Through deliberate practice, you are able to make steady progress in improving your piano playing skills, and you are able to see the results of your effort through improved performance and accuracy over time.

Effectiveness of practice

There are several factors that can influence the effectiveness of practice in motor skill acquisition and retention:

1. Frequency and duration of practice: The frequency and duration of practice sessions can impact the effectiveness of practice. Consistent and regular practice is generally more effective than infrequent or sporadic practice.

2. Type of practice: The type of practice used can also impact effectiveness. Deliberate practice, which involves focused and intentional practice sessions, is generally more effective than unfocused or random practice.

3. Feedback: Feedback during practice sessions is essential for learners to adjust their movements, correct errors, and reinforce correct movements. Immediate and specific feedback is generally more effective than delayed or general feedback.

Chapter 2: Motor learning

4. Motivation and engagement: Learners who are motivated and engaged in their practice sessions are more likely to see improvements in their skill acquisition and retention. Setting goals, providing challenges, and making practice sessions interesting and enjoyable can all enhance motivation and engagement.

5. Skill level: The effectiveness of practice can also depend on the learner's skill level. Beginners may benefit from more frequent and varied practice, while advanced learners may require more targeted and specific practice to continue improving.

6. Environment: The environment in which practice takes place can also impact its effectiveness. A well-lit and spacious practice area with appropriate equipment can enhance learning and skill acquisition.

7. Rest and recovery: Adequate rest and recovery time between practice sessions is essential for learners to consolidate their learning and retain motor skills over time. Overtraining or fatigue can lead to reduced effectiveness and even injury.

By considering these factors and designing practice sessions accordingly, learners can maximize the effectiveness of their practice and improve their motor skill acquisition and retention.

ENVIRONMENTAL FACTORS

Environmental factors such as equipment, coaching, and social support can have a significant impact on motor learning and development.

Equipment

The type and quality of equipment available can influence an individual's motor learning and development. High-quality equipment that is appropriate for the individual's skill level and needs can facilitate motor skill acquisition and enhance performance. For example, using appropriate footwear and equipment in sports can reduce the risk of injury and improve performance.

Coaching

The quality and style of coaching can also affect motor learning and development. Effective coaches can provide feedback, instruction, and motivation that can enhance skill acquisition and help individuals reach their full potential. Coaches who use a positive and supportive approach can also promote confidence and self-efficacy, which can improve performance and promote continued engagement in physical activity.

Social support

The social environment in which an individual learns and develops motor skills can also have a significant impact on their progress. Supportive social networks can provide motivation, encouragement, and feedback that can enhance skill acquisition and promote continued engagement in physical activity. Additionally, social support can help individuals develop a sense of belonging and connection to others, which can positively impact their mental health and wellbeing.

By providing appropriate equipment, effective coaching, and supportive social environments, individuals can enhance their motor skills, improve their performance, and promote their physical and mental wellbeing.

SPECIAL POPULATIONS

Motor learning in children, older adults and individuals with disabilities

Motor learning principles can be applied to special populations such as children, older adults, and individuals with disabilities to improve their motor skill acquisition and development. However, the specific considerations and adaptations required to effectively apply these principles may vary depending on the population in question.

1. Children: When applying motor learning principles to children, it is important to consider their developmental stage and adjust teaching strategies accordingly. Children may require more frequent and explicit feedback, shorter practice sessions, and a more playful approach to learning. Additionally, incorporating visual and auditory cues and providing opportunities for exploration and creativity can be effective for promoting motor skill development in children.

2. Older adults: As individuals age, their ability to learn and acquire new motor skills may be affected by factors such as decreased physical ability, changes in cognitive function, and increased risk of injury. When working with older adults, it may be helpful to incorporate lower intensity activities, longer rest periods, and more explicit instructions to facilitate learning. Additionally, focusing on functional movements that improve daily living skills can be effective for promoting motor skill development in older adults.

3. Individuals with disabilities: Individuals with disabilities may face unique challenges when learning and developing motor skills, and adaptations may be required to effectively apply motor learning principles. Depending on the individual's specific disability, modifications to equipment or teaching strategies may be necessary. Additionally, incorporating multisensory feedback and breaking down complex movements into smaller, more manageable steps can be

effective for promoting motor skill development in individuals with disabilities.

Therefore, motor learning principles can be applied to special populations such as children, older adults, and individuals with disabilities to promote motor skill acquisition and development. However, adaptations and modifications may be necessary to effectively apply these principles in these populations. By considering the unique needs and characteristics of each population, individuals can create more inclusive and effective environments for skill development.

Motor development, control, and rehabilitation in specific populations

It is important to consider motor learning principles when working with children, older adults, and individuals with disabilities, as these populations may have unique needs and challenges related to their motor development, motor control, and rehabilitation.

1. In children, motor learning principles can help to promote the development of fundamental movement skills, which are critical for physical activity participation and overall health and wellbeing. By using appropriate teaching strategies and providing opportunities for practice and feedback, children can develop strong motor skills and improve their movement efficiency and accuracy.

2. In older adults, motor learning principles can be applied to promote functional movement and independence, which can improve quality of life and reduce the risk of falls and other injuries. By incorporating appropriate modifications and adjustments, older adults can improve their motor control and reduce the impact of age-related declines in physical function.
3. In individuals with disabilities, motor learning principles can be used to facilitate rehabilitation and improve functional outcomes. By adapting teaching strategies and incorporating appropriate equipment and modifications, individuals with disabilities can improve their motor control and movement patterns, enhancing their ability to perform daily living tasks and participate in physical activity.

Therefore, considering motor learning principles in these populations can lead to improved motor development, motor control, and rehabilitation outcomes, promoting physical activity participation, overall health, and quality of life.

APPLICATIONS

Real-world settings

Motor learning principles can be applied in real-world settings, such as sports, physical therapy, and occupational therapy, to improve skill acquisition and performance. Here are some specific

Chapter 2: Motor learning

examples of how motor learning principles can be applied in these settings:

1. Sports training: Coaches and trainers can use motor learning principles to improve athletes' performance and skill acquisition. Deliberate practice, variable practice, and feedback are commonly used motor learning principles in sports training. For example, by providing specific feedback and incorporating different practice conditions, athletes can improve their motor skills and enhance their ability to perform under pressure. Additionally, coaches can use video feedback and analysis to help athletes visualize and correct movement patterns.

2. Physical therapy: In physical therapy, motor learning principles can be used to help patients recover from injury or illness. The principles of repetition, variability, and feedback are important in this setting. By providing patients with opportunities for practice, adjusting task difficulty, and providing feedback on performance, patients can improve their motor control and enhance their recovery.

3. Occupational therapy: Occupational therapists can use motor learning principles to improve patients' ability to perform everyday tasks. For example, therapists can use task-specific training to help patients learn the skills necessary for specific job tasks. Additionally, therapists can use feedback and coaching to help patients learn new motor patterns and improve their movement efficiency.

Overall, motor learning principles can be applied in a variety of real-world settings to improve skill acquisition and performance. By incorporating appropriate teaching strategies, practice conditions, and feedback, individuals can improve their motor skills and enhance their ability to perform in a variety of contexts, whether it is in sports, physical therapy, or occupational therapy.

Here are some case studies that illustrate the application of motor learning principles in real-world settings:

1. Sports training: In a study of collegiate basketball players, researchers used motor learning principles to improve shooting accuracy. Specifically, the athletes were randomly assigned to either a blocked practice group (repeating the same shot type over and over) or a random practice group (shooting different types of shots in a random order). The random practice group showed greater improvement in shooting accuracy compared to the blocked practice group, suggesting that variability in practice conditions can enhance motor learning. (Mihara et al., 2012)

2. Physical therapy: In a study of patients with stroke-related hemiparesis, researchers used motor learning principles to improve walking ability. The patients received task-specific training, which involved practicing walking on a treadmill while receiving feedback on their gait pattern. The researchers found that the patients showed significant improvements in walking

speed and stride length after completing the training, suggesting that repetition and feedback can enhance motor learning in patients with neurological impairments. (Reisman et al., 2013)

3. Occupational therapy: In a case study of a patient with Parkinson's disease, an occupational therapist used motor learning principles to improve the patient's ability to perform self-care tasks. The therapist provided the patient with structured practice sessions, including breaking down the task into smaller components and providing feedback on performance. The patient showed significant improvement in their ability to perform the task after completing the training, suggesting that practice and feedback can enhance motor learning even in patients with degenerative neurological conditions. (Taylor et al., 2012)

These case studies illustrate how motor learning principles can be applied in real-world settings to improve skill acquisition and performance in a variety of contexts, including sports, physical therapy, and occupational therapy. By incorporating appropriate teaching strategies, practice conditions, and feedback, individuals can improve their motor skills and enhance their ability to perform in a variety of contexts.

Examples

Examples of how motor learning principles can be used to improve motor skill performance and enhance quality of life

1. Parkinson's disease: People with Parkinson's disease often experience motor deficits, such as tremors and bradykinesia. Motor learning principles, such as intensive practice, can help improve motor skill performance and reduce motor deficits in these individuals. For example, studies have shown that people with Parkinson's disease who engage in intensive practice of balance and gait tasks can improve their performance and reduce their risk of falls (Keus et al., 2007).

2. Stroke: Stroke survivors often experience motor deficits, such as hemiparesis and impaired motor control. Motor learning principles, such as task-specific training and feedback, can help improve motor skill performance and enhance quality of life in these individuals. For example, studies have shown that stroke survivors who receive task-specific training on activities of daily living, such as dressing and bathing, can improve their performance and enhance their ability to live independently (Lang et al., 2008).

3. Autism spectrum disorder (ASD): People with ASD often experience motor deficits, such as poor coordination and balance. Motor learning principles, such as variability in practice and feedback, can help improve motor skill performance and enhance quality of life in these individuals.

For example, studies have shown that children with ASD who engage in activities that involve variability in motor demands, such as playing sports, can improve their motor coordination and social skills (Pan, 2010).

Overall, motor learning principles can be used to improve motor skill performance and enhance quality of life in a variety of populations, including those with Parkinson's disease, stroke, and ASD. By incorporating appropriate teaching strategies, practice conditions, and feedback, individuals can improve their motor skills and enhance their ability to perform in a variety of contexts, which can have a positive impact on their overall well-being.

Motor control and sport performance

Motor control plays a crucial role in sport performance. Motor skills are essential for athletes to perform complex movements with accuracy, speed, and efficiency. Motor skills can be acquired through practice and repetition, and they can be refined through feedback and deliberate practice.

Motor skills are learned through a process of motor learning, which involves several stages. The first stage is the cognitive stage, where the athlete is introduced to the movement and must learn the basic motor patterns. The second stage is the associative stage, where the athlete refines the movement and makes adjustments to improve performance. The final stage is the autonomous stage, where the athlete can perform the movement without conscious effort.

Athletic performance is heavily influenced by motor control, as it determines the quality and efficiency of movements. For example, in running, motor control plays a significant role in maintaining proper form and optimizing stride length and frequency. In basketball, motor control is essential for shooting accuracy and ball handling.

Athletes can improve their motor control and performance through a variety of methods, including:

1. Practice and repetition: Consistent and deliberate practice is essential for acquiring and refining motor skills.
2. Feedback: Feedback from coaches or trainers can provide athletes with information about their performance and help them make adjustments to improve their motor control.
3. Visualization: Mental rehearsal and visualization can help athletes improve their motor control by mentally rehearsing movements before executing them.
4. Strength and conditioning: Improving strength and conditioning can enhance motor control by increasing muscular control and coordination.

Therefore, motor control plays a critical role in sport performance by determining the quality and efficiency of movements. Motor skills are acquired through practice and repetition and can be refined through feedback and deliberate practice. Improving motor control can enhance athletic performance and help athletes achieve their full potential.

Motor control in older people

Motor control plays a critical role in older adults' performance, particularly in the areas of mobility, balance, and activities of daily living. As we age, changes occur in the nervous system, musculoskeletal system, and sensory systems, which can lead to declines in motor control and functional performance.

Motor skills in older adults can be acquired and refined through exercise, practice, and rehabilitation programs. These programs can help to maintain or improve muscle strength, joint mobility, balance, and coordination. Additionally, training in specific activities, such as walking or stair climbing, can improve the specific motor skills required for those activities.

Motor control has a significant impact on older adults' functional performance, which is critical for maintaining independence and quality of life. Declines in motor control can lead to increased risk of falls, difficulty performing activities of daily living, and decreased mobility. Conversely, improvements in motor control can lead to increased independence, improved quality of life, and reduced risk of falls and other adverse outcomes.

There are several interventions and strategies that can help to improve motor control in older adults:

1. Exercise: Regular exercise, particularly strength and balance training, can improve muscle strength, balance, and coordination, leading to improved motor control and functional performance.

2. Rehabilitation: Rehabilitation programs, such as physical therapy or occupational therapy, can help to improve specific motor skills and functional performance.

3. Assistive devices: The use of assistive devices, such as canes or walkers, can improve stability and mobility, leading to improved motor control and functional performance.

4. Environmental modifications: Modifications to the environment, such as removing trip hazards or adding handrails, can improve safety and mobility, leading to improved motor control and functional performance.

In conclusion, motor control plays a critical role in older adults' functional performance, particularly in the areas of mobility, balance, and activities of daily living. Motor skills can be acquired and refined through exercise, practice, and rehabilitation programs, leading to improved functional performance and quality of life. Interventions and strategies that improve motor control can help older adults maintain their independence and reduce their risk of falls and other adverse outcomes.

CHAPTER 3: CORTEX

SOMATOMOTOR CORTEX AND VOLUNTARY MOVEMENT

The somatomotor cortex consists of the primary motor cortex, association motor cortex, and frontal eye field (Fig. 3.1). All three areas can be identified on the lateral side of the brain and extend to the medial side of the brain hemisphere.

Cortical Motor Neural Mapping

The neurons of the cortex accumulate together according to their similarities in function, shape, and size, then form a *cortical cell column*. The size of the cortical column can be about 5 mm in diameter when viewed from the brain's surface.

The primary motor cortex lies just anterior to the central sulcus. The primary motor cortex is also called M1, Brodmann's area 4, or the precentral gyrus.

The association motor cortex is also named Brodmann's area 6 and lies anterior to the primary motor cortex (Fig. 3.2). Brodmann's area 6 can be seen on both the lateral and medial sides of the brain hemisphere. The part on the lateral side of the brain hemisphere is called the premotor cortex, while the part on the medial side is called the association motor cortex. As described later, the premotor and association motor cortex functions are different in controlling voluntary movements.

The frontal eye field is also called Brodmann's area 8 and lies anterior to the upper part of the premotor cortex. The function of the frontal eye field is related to the control and coordination of voluntary eye movement.

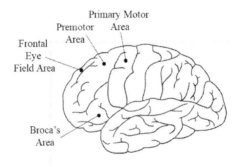

Figure 3.1. They are the primary motor area, association motor areas, and frontal eye field.

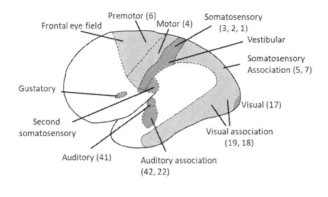

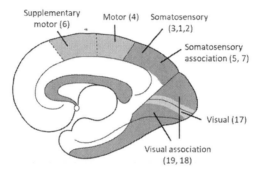

Figure 3.2. Cortical surface locations of motor control areas.
Primary motor (4), premotor (6), primary somatosensory (3, 2, 1), somatosensory association (5, 7), visual (17) and visual association cortices. The numbers are Brodmann brain areas.

One muscle has more than one cortical column to supply.

In the primary motor cortex, it has been demonstrated that more than one cortical column can innervate a lower motor neuron in the spinal cord (Fig. 3.3). This means that one muscle is supplied by more than one cortical cell column.

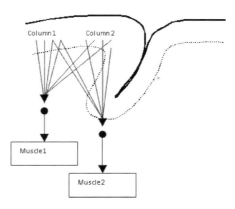

Figure 3.3. Connections between the cortical motor neurons and muscles of the hand. Figure (above) shows an example of the connections between the cortical motor neurons and muscles of the hand. It demonstrates that one muscle is supplied by more than one cortical cell column.

One cortical area (colony) can supply more than one muscle.

The cortex has a mixed pattern of functional cortical colonies controlling different muscles (Fig. 3.4). There is no simple correlation of one-to-one between the cortical area and the muscles. For example, the cortical colony supplying the fingers can be found in the cortical area controlling the muscles for wrist extension. Thus, describing a cortical area regulating a muscle rather than a one-to-one relationship is more appropriate. Predominant supply from the motor cortex to the muscle gives the overall organization of somatotopic motor representation, which forms the homunculus.

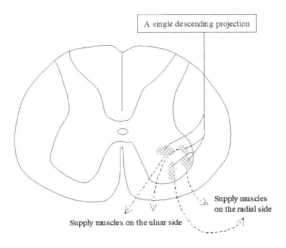

Figure 3.4. The above figure shows that a single descending project can synapse on four different lower motor neurons in the anterior horn of the spinal cord. The upper two groups of lower motor neurons of the spinal cord supply the muscles on the ulnar side of the arm. The lower two groups of neurons supply the muscles on the radial side of the arm.

Hot Spot in the Motor Control

Only one group of cortical neurons has a low threshold for a particular muscle. This group of cells is called a *hot spot*. The hot spot supplies a single muscle most sensitive to stimulation (Fig. 3.5).

As mentioned earlier, numerous neurons from a relatively large cortical area can supply a single muscle. However, the thresholds for initiating muscle action are different among these neurons. In other words, some neurons are more sensitive to inducing specific muscle activation than others. This has been demonstrated by intracortical microstimulation. Therefore, they form an essential basis, contributing to the primary motor cortex's dominant areas that control voluntary movement. For example, stimulation of the middle third of the primary motor cortex induces muscle contraction in the arm. However, when we examine the detailed somatotopic organization of this area, one group of neurons is most sensitive in causing wrist extension.

The group of neurons mentioned above is not the only one that can induce wrist extension. Other neurons, for example, those that are 3 mm away from this group, can also generate wrist extension. Still, higher strength and a longer duration of stimulation are needed to induce the same degree of wrist extension. Similarly, the cortical area supplying the shoulder muscles can also facilitate thumb muscle activation. Therefore, the cortical map providing voluntary muscles has a mixed pattern. This means that a group of neurons predominantly controls a particular group of muscles in a region (for example, the wrist muscles). Still, they can also facilitate the muscles of other regions (for example, the finger muscles), but with less sensitivity.

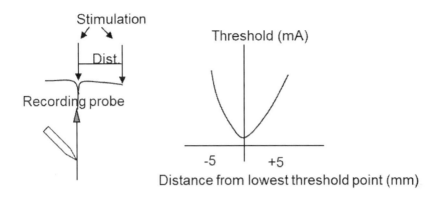

Figure 3.5. The distance between cortical areas induces the single-fiber activity of the pyramidal tract. The above figure shows that the distance between cortical areas induces the single-fiber activity of the pyramidal tract. Higher stimulation is needed when the electrode is away from the neuron. Excitatory postsynaptic potential (EPSP) is greater in the neurons supplying distal muscles than in the neurons supplying proximal muscles (Andersen et al., 1975).

Patterns of pyramidal neurons control agonist and antagonist muscles.

The figure below (Fig. 3.6) shows the patterns of connections between M1 neurons and neurons in the anterior horn of the spinal cord.

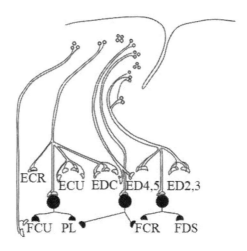

Figure 3.6. The patterns of connections between M1 neurons and neurons in the anterior horn of the spinal cord. The above figure shows the patterns of pyramidal tract neurons controlling agonist and antagonist muscles of the wrist muscles. Here, the top row represents the extensors, e.g., extensor carpi radialis and ulnaris (ECR, ECU). The bottom row represents the flexor muscles, e.g., flexor carpi ulnaris and flexor carpi radialis (FCU, FCR).

(1) Pyramidal tract neurons project to the agonist muscles. This group of neurons is involved in the initiation of the prime mover.

(2) Dual projection of pyramidal tract neurons. A single pyramidal tract neuron can branch and project to both agonist and antagonist muscles. It forms the basis of one pyramidal neuron facilitating the agonist muscle and simultaneously suppressing the antagonist muscles.

(3) Pyramidal tract neurons project to the antagonist muscles only. This group of neurons is involved in suppressing a single group of muscles.

As seen in performing muscle contractions, it is necessary to facilitate the agonist muscles and simultaneously suppress the antagonist muscles. For example, activation of a neuron supplying the forearm region can induce muscle activity of flexor pollicis brevis and, at the same time, inhibit flexor carpi ulnaris. This will allow the action of flexing the thumb to be achieved.

Presetting, Precision, and Orientation

Human voluntary movement involves presetting, precision, and orientation. Studies have shown that the pyramidal tract neuron plays an essential role in presetting, precision, and orientation of the voluntary movement. However, pyramidal tract neurons are not necessary to provide force.

Presetting of Voluntary Movement

The presetting of voluntary movement is a process in which the brain prepares for a voluntary movement before it actually occurs. This involves a series of neural processes that occur seconds before the action is initiated.

A critical aspect of the presetting of voluntary movement is the preparation of the motor cortex, which is a region of the brain responsible for initiating and controlling voluntary movements. Studies have shown that the motor cortex can become active several seconds before a voluntary movement occurs, indicating that the brain is preparing for the movement in advance.

Another important aspect of the presetting of voluntary movement is the involvement of the cerebellum, which plays a key role in coordinating voluntary movements and maintaining balance and posture. The cerebellum receives input from the motor cortex and other parts of the brain, and uses this information to predict the movements that will be required and to adjust the movement as needed.

In addition to these neural processes, the presetting of voluntary movement also involves preparatory movements, such as shifting weight or adjusting posture, that help to position the body for the upcoming movement. These preparatory movements can occur in advance of the voluntary movement and can help to optimize the efficiency and accuracy of the movement.

Overall, the presetting of voluntary movement is an important aspect of motor control that allows the brain to prepare for and optimize voluntary movements. Understanding the neural and behavioral processes involved in this phenomenon can provide insights into the underlying mechanisms of motor control and may lead to the development of new strategies for optimizing motor performance.

The pyramidal tract neuron is involved in the presetting activity in reflex circuits before movement. As demonstrated in monkey studies, pyramidal tract neuronal activity occurs before voluntary action. The relationship between the pyramidal tract neurons and EMG (electromyography) activity is also established. Experiments have demonstrated that pyramidal tract neuronal activity is seen before EMG activity. A trained monkey was given visual instructions for action. The EMG activity could be recorded in the wrist extensor muscles to correlate it with the visual signals and pyramidal tract neuronal activity. The sequence of events was recorded as visual stimulation–induced pyramidal tract neuronal activity, followed by EMG activity, and then the onset of muscle movement. This event indicates that pyramidal tract neurons in the somatomotor cortex are involved in presetting movement action.

Force

The pyramidal tract neurons respond to changes in contraction force demands. For example, if you put a brick in your hand, the pyramidal tract neurons will be activated; however, if you do elbow flexion, the pyramidal tract neurons are not sensitive to the power changes.

Precision

Pyramidal tract neurons fire more at precision movement, such as distal (finger) motor activation. They are sensitive to finger precision grip but are insensitive to force requirements. Similarly, pyramidal tract neurons show low activity in hand (not finger) power grip.

The regulation of movement precision refers to the mechanisms and processes that enable the body to execute specific movements with a high degree of accuracy and consistency. This involves the integration of sensory, neural, and muscular processes, as well as feedback mechanisms to adjust and refine the movement in real-time.

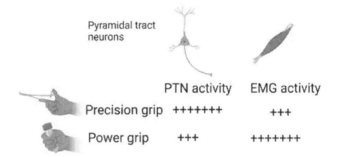

Figure 3.7. Pyramidal tract neuronal (PTN) activity in primary motor cortex during precision grip and power grip.
The PTN activity increases when performing a precision grip; however, PTN is low when performing a power grip. Electromyograph (EMG) shows the muscle activity which is greater in the power grip task.

Chapter 3: Cortex

The regulation of movement precision is achieved through the following mechanisms:

1. Sensory feedback: The brain receives information about the environment and body position from muscle and joint receptors. This feedback is used to adjust and refine the movement in real-time, ensuring that the movement is executed with high precision.
2. Motor planning: The primary motor cortex generates a motor plan that specifies the precise movement needed to achieve a particular goal. This plan includes information about the degree of force, timing, and duration of muscle contractions needed to execute the movement precisely.
3. Neural coordination: The basal ganglia and cerebellum coordinate and refine movement. These brain regions help to ensure that the appropriate muscles are activated at the right time and with the right amount of force to execute the movement with precision.
4. Muscle control: The muscles must contract and relax in a coordinated manner to produce the desired movement. The degree of force, timing, and duration of muscle contractions is tightly controlled to ensure that the movement is executed precisely and accurately.
5. Feedback mechanisms: Muscle spindles and other sensory receptors provide feedback to the brain about the position and

movement of the body. This feedback is used to adjust and refine the motor plan in real-time, ensuring that the movement is executed with the highest degree of precision and accuracy possible.

In summary, the regulation of movement precision involves a complex and highly coordinated process that integrates various sensory, neural, and muscular processes to achieve a specific goal. It requires the ability to adjust and refine movements in real-time based on sensory feedback, and it is essential for many daily activities that require a high level of skill and training to master.

Orientation

Pyramidal tract neurons are essential in determining movement orientation. They are directionally selective and have strength in the cellular firing rate of the preferred movement direction.

The population vector of pyramidal tract neurons shows that groups of cells represent the direction of movement encoded in the neurons. The population vector is used to predict the direction of motion. For any given direction of action, the direction vectors of the individual cells can be combined to yield a population vector, reflecting the strength of the cells' response during the movement.

Pyramidal tract neurons represent all directions of movement.

A single neuron can be active during movement in various directions. However, neurons fire best when the movement is in a preferred direction, for example, moving the thumb upward. Furthermore, the preferred orientation is not the same among different neurons. For example, one neuron fires more when the thumb is to be moved downward, although it also fires when the movement is in other directions. Therefore, in combination, all directions of movement are covered by the pyramidal tract neurons.

Spike-Triggered Averaging

Activation of a single pyramidal tract neuron can induce an output assembly of various activated motor neural pathways, which, in turn, activate one or more muscles (Fig. 3.8). At the same time, this can also inhibit one or more muscles. In this manner, the muscles activated or inhibited by the pyramidal tract neurons largely depend upon functional needs.

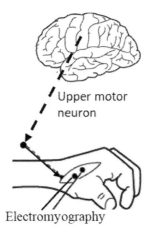

Figure 3.8. Instructions for precision grip. The above figure shows instructions for precision grip, single pyramidal tract neuron (PTN) induced multi-EMG activities of hand muscle.

Plasticity of the Cortical Motor Map

Studies have shown that the brain cortex can rapidly reorganize itself after removing its target muscle. The reorganization of the cortical map can occur quickly, even within sixty minutes of a muscle lesion.

Researchers have demonstrated that the primary motor cortex can reorganize the cortical map after transecting the buccal and mandibular branches of the facial nerve, which supply the orbicular oris. After this transection, the primary motor cortex supplying the orbicularis oris (vibrissa muscles) changes to supply the forelimb and periocular muscles. It means that the cortical neurons have

Chapter 3: Cortex

reorganized their supply of target organs. This hypothesis is further supported by examining the EMG activity of the muscle. As shown, the forearm muscles (wrist extensors) receive projections from the cortical area, which previously supplied the orbicularis oris. After buccal and mandibular nerve transection, these neurons change to supply the forearm muscles.

The GABAergic interneurons may be a critical element in shaping the pattern of cortical connections (Fig. 3.9).

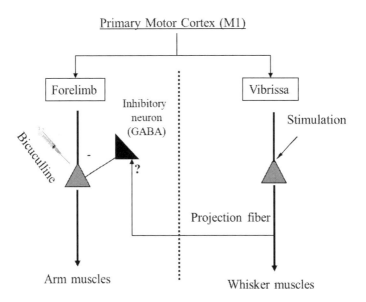

Figure 3.9. Proposed working model for reorganizing the cortical motor map. The above figure shows a proposed working model for reorganizing the cortical motor map. It indicates that

GABAergic neurons play an inhibitory role between the two pyramidal tract neurons from different areas. Conversely, the GABA antagonist (bicuculline) has inhibitory effects on one motor neuron (here it is the vibrissa), activating the neuron supplying another (forelimb) muscle.

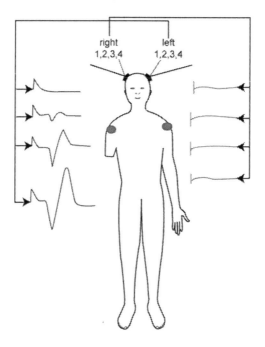

Figure 3.10. Cortical map plasticity in humans. The human cortex reorganizing its motor map after target organ damage. The above figure shows how the human cortex can reorganize its motor map after target organ damage. For example, a person had a right arm amputation about four years ago. The researcher showed that stimulation at the points on the scalp elicits EMG

activity in the deltoid muscles. However, EMG activity in the deltoid differs between the left and right sides. The right deltoid muscle (lesion side) receives a much higher response revealed by EMG activity than the left deltoid muscle (intact side). This suggests that the deltoid muscle on the lesion side gets a much greater supply from the brain areas than the intact side. This means that the cortex supplies to the right arm have reorganized to supply the deltoid muscle following the amputation of the right arm. Therefore, human studies support that the human cortex can also reorganize its cortical motor map after a peripheral muscle lesion.

ASSOCIATION MOTOR CORTEX

The association motor cortex is a region of the brain that plays a key role in motor planning and control. It is located in the frontal lobe of the brain, adjacent to the primary motor cortex (M1), and is composed of several sub-regions, including the premotor cortex (PM) and the supplementary motor area (SMA).

The association motor cortex is involved in a range of motor functions, including the planning and execution of voluntary movements, as well as the integration of sensory feedback to adjust movements in real-time. It receives input from other brain regions, including the basal ganglia and cerebellum, and sends output to subcortical regions involved in motor control, such as the spinal cord and brainstem.

Lesions in the association motor cortex can lead to a range of motor deficits, including apraxia, which is the inability to perform purposeful movements despite intact motor function. Additionally, disruptions in the association motor cortex have been linked to movement disorders, such as Parkinson's disease and dystonia.

Overall, the association motor cortex plays a critical role in motor control and is essential for the planning, execution, and adjustment of movements in response to sensory feedback and task demands.

The areas of the association motor cortex lie near the primary motor cortex and play an important role in performing visual and internally guided movements. The association motor cortex is not directly involved in the execution of voluntary movement, but it is involved in motor planning. In the following section, we will focus on the description of motor planning by the association motor cortex and its correlation with other brain parts.

Anatomy

Premotor Cortex

The *premotor cortex* (PM) lies in the lateral part of Brodmann's area 6 and is anterior to the primary motor cortex. It has no Betz cells (no large pyramidal neurons in layer V).

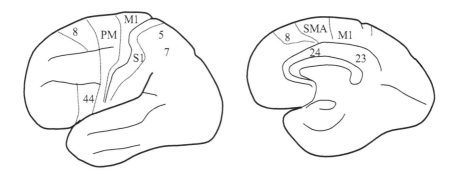

Figure 3.11. Association areas of somatomotor and somatosensory cortices of the human brain. The above figure shows association areas of somatomotor and somatosensory cortices of the human brain. Here, the drawing on the left is a lateral view of the brain. Furthermore, the picture on the right depicts a medial view of the brain. Abbreviations: PM: premotor cortex; M1: primary motor cortex; S1: primary sensory cortex; SMA: supplementary motor cortical area; Brodmann's areas 5, 7, 8, 23, 24, and 44.

Supplementary Motor Area

The *supplementary motor area* (SMA) is in the medial part of Brodmann's area 6, which is on the medial side, above the cingulate cortex, and anterior to the primary motor cortex (Fig. 3.11).

Broca's Area 44

Broca's area 44 is a region of the brain located in the left hemisphere of the frontal lobe, specifically in the posterior part of the inferior frontal gyrus (Fig. 3.11). It is named after Paul Broca, a French physician who first described its role in language production in the 19th century.

Broca's area 44 is primarily involved in the production of speech and language. Specifically, it is responsible for the planning and execution of the movements necessary for speech production, such as the movements of the lips, tongue, and vocal cords. Damage to Broca's area can result in a type of language impairment called Broca's aphasia, which is characterized by difficulty with language production while language comprehension remains intact.

In addition to its role in language production, Broca's area 44 has also been implicated in a variety of other cognitive processes, including working memory, attention, and social cognition. Recent studies have suggested that Broca's area may play a role in the processing of hierarchical structures, such as those found in music and mathematics.

Cingulate cortex

The cingulate motor cortex (CMC) is a region of the brain that is located in the anterior cingulate cortex, a part of the frontal lobe (Brodmann's area 23 and 24). It is involved in the planning, initiation, and execution of voluntary movements, and works in conjunction with other motor regions of the brain, such as the primary motor cortex and premotor cortex.

Motor dysfunction can occur when there is damage to the cingulate motor cortex, which can result in a range of movement disorders. For example, damage to the CMC has been associated with difficulties in initiating movements, impaired motor coordination, and muscle weakness.

One example of a movement disorder that can be associated with dysfunction in the cingulate motor cortex is apraxia, a condition in which individuals have difficulty performing purposeful movements, despite having intact motor abilities. In some cases of apraxia, the CMC has been identified as a key area of damage.

Understanding the role of the cingulate motor cortex in motor function is important for developing treatments for movement disorders, as well as for gaining insights into the complex neural mechanisms underlying movement control in the brain.

Frontal eys field

The frontal eye field (FEF) is a region of the brain located in the frontal lobe, specifically in the superior frontal gyrus (Brodmann's area 8). It plays an important role in the control of eye movements and visual attention.

The FEF is involved in the initiation of voluntary eye movements, including saccades (rapid eye movements between two fixation points) and smooth pursuit movements (tracking of a moving object with the eyes). It is also involved in the suppression of reflexive eye movements, such as those triggered by a sudden change in visual input.

The FEF is thought to work in concert with other regions of the brain, including the primary motor cortex and the supplementary motor area, to plan and execute voluntary movements. Damage to the FEF can result in deficits in eye movement control, as well as impairments in motor planning and execution.

Overall, the FEF is an important region of the brain that plays a crucial role in the control of eye movements and other motor functions. Understanding its function is important for understanding the complex neural mechanisms underlying motor control in the brain.

Brodmann's areas 5 and 7

Brodmann's areas 5 and 7 are regions of the brain that are located in the parietal lobe, and they play important roles in motor control.

Area 5, also known as the superior parietal lobule, is involved in the integration of sensory information from multiple modalities, including proprioception, touch, and vision, to form a unified representation of the body and the external environment. This information is used to guide movements, such as reaching and grasping, by providing information about the location of objects in space and the position of the body.

Area 7, also known as the inferior parietal lobule, is involved in the processing of visual and somatosensory information related to spatial orientation and attention. This region is important for spatial perception and awareness of the body in space, and it is involved in the planning and execution of movements that require spatial orientation, such as walking and navigating through a complex environment.

Areas 5 and 7 are closely interconnected, and together they form a network of brain regions that are involved in motor planning and execution. These regions are thought to work together to integrate sensory information with motor commands, allowing for accurate and coordinated movements.

Damage to areas 5 and 7 can result in deficits in spatial perception, coordination, and motor planning, leading to impairments in movements such as reaching and grasping, walking, and navigating through space.

Overall, areas 5 and 7 are critical brain regions for motor control, playing important roles in integrating sensory information with motor commands to guide movements and maintain spatial orientation. Therefore, lesions to areas 5 and 7 will cause a reluctance to use the contralateral arm and hand. As a result, the patient often neglects the opposite side of the body.

Chapter 3: Cortex

Connections of the Association Motor Cortex

The association motor cortical area has wide connections with many other brain areas. Below, we describe the major connections of the association motor cortex with other cortical areas, the subcortical regions, and the brainstem.

Cortico-Cortical Connections: The association motor cortex has broad connections with other motor-related areas. As seen in the below figure, reciprocal links between primary and association motor and sensory areas are found.

Corticostriatal and Corticobulbar Projections: The association motor cortex has strong connections to the thalamus that, in turn, connect to the basal ganglia. The association motor cortex has rich connections with brainstem structures such as the red nucleus, substantia nigra, reticular formation, and vestibular nucleus. All these tracts project to both sides of the body and are involved in the complex nature of voluntary movement.

Corticospinal Projections: The association motor cortex contributes largely (about 40%) to the corticospinal tract. The corticospinal tract is the major descending projection for voluntary movement.

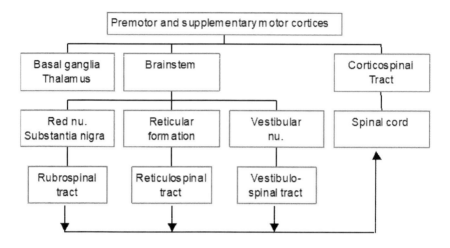

Figure 3.12. Summary. A flowchart summarizes the projections from the association somatomotor cortex to the subcortex, brainstem, and spinal cord.

Stimulation of the Association Motor Cortex

Electrical stimulation of the association motor cortex can induce skeletal muscle contraction. Compared with the electrical stimulation of M1 neurons (the neurons in the primary motor cortex), higher intensities of electrical current stimulation to the association motor cortex are needed to produce skeletal muscle contraction. Furthermore, a long duration of stimulation is required for the association motor cortex to produce muscle contraction.

Association Motor Cortical Map

Premotor cortex (PM): There is no precise localization pattern of motor representation in the premotor cortex. The axial and proximal muscles are represented from the rostral to the caudal direction in the association motor cortical map. The head area representation is at the inferior, and the tail area representation is at the superior. The premotor cortex is involved in performing visually guided movement and is also responsible for visual orientation-required movement. This means that the premotor cortex executes movement direction signaled by visual instruction.

Supplementary motor area (SMA): There is no precise localization pattern of motor representation in the supplementary motor area. A general order of motor representation is that the face is in the rostral part, and the leg is in the caudal part of the supplementary motor area. Furthermore, the proximal part of the body is in the dorsal region, and the distal part is in the ventral part of the supplementary motor area.

Data concerning the cortical motor map is mainly derived from studies of experimental animals. Human primary and association motor cortices appear similar to cortical motor organization found in experimental animals. Studies have shown that electrical stimulation of M1 neurons induces muscle twitches in the contralateral part of the body, and there is no occurrence of complex movements when M1 is stimulated. However, stimulation of the human supplementary motor area induces complex movement. Furthermore, premotor cortex stimulation induces head and eye movements and trunk turning.

Externally Guided Movement

Externally guided movements are movements that are guided by external cues or stimuli in the environment. These cues can be visual, auditory, or tactile, and they provide information about the location, timing, and direction of the movement. Examples of externally guided movements include reaching for an object, catching a ball, or following a moving target.

When performing an externally guided movement, the brain processes sensory information from the external environment and uses this information to generate motor commands that control the movement. The sensory information is initially processed in primary sensory areas of the brain, such as the visual cortex for visual stimuli or the somatosensory cortex for tactile stimuli. This information is then transmitted to the premotor cortex, which integrates the sensory information with motor commands and generates the appropriate movement.

The generation of externally guided movements typically involves a combination of feedforward and feedback mechanisms. Feedforward mechanisms involve the prediction of the movement based on the available sensory information, allowing for the

Chapter 3: Cortex

movement to be initiated before the external cue is actually encountered. Feedback mechanisms involve the continuous monitoring of the movement and the use of sensory feedback to make adjustments to the movement as necessary.

Externally guided movements are essential for many activities of daily living and are commonly used in sports and other physical activities.

The premotor cortex is a region of the brain located in the frontal lobe, anterior to the primary motor cortex, and it plays an important role in the planning and execution of movements. In particular, the premotor cortex is involved in the generation of movements that are guided by external cues or stimuli, such as those involved in externally guided movements.

The premotor cortex (PM) receives input from the association visual cortex and other sensory areas of the brain, allowing it to process information about the location, timing, and direction of external cues. This information is used to generate motor commands that control the movement. The premotor cortex is also involved in the generation of feedforward mechanisms that allow for the movement to be initiated before the external cue is actually encountered.

Overall, the premotor cortex plays an important role in the generation of externally guided movements by integrating sensory information with motor commands and generating the appropriate movement. Dysfunction of the premotor cortex can lead to deficits in the planning and execution of movements, highlighting the important role of this brain region in motor control.

Internally guided movement

Internally guided movements are movements that are generated based on internal cues, such as an individual's intentions, goals, and memories, rather than external cues from the environment. These movements are self-initiated and do not require external stimuli to be generated.

In internally guided movements, the motor commands for the movement are generated in the absence of sensory feedback from the environment. Instead, the brain generates these commands based on internal representations of the desired movement, which are stored in memory and accessed when needed. These internal representations may be based on previous experiences or motor plans that have been developed through practice or learning.

Internally guided movements are essential for many activities of daily living, such as reaching for a cup or walking to a destination. They also play an important role in complex actions, such as playing a musical instrument or performing a dance routine, which require precise control and coordination of multiple movements.

The generation of internally guided movements involves a combination of brain regions, including the supplementary motor area as well as others such as premotor cortex, and basal ganglia.

These regions work together to generate motor commands based on internal cues and to coordinate and control the movements.

Overall, internally guided movements are an important aspect of motor control, allowing individuals to generate movements based on their own goals and intentions rather than external cues from the environment.

Supplementary motor area

The supplementary motor area (SMA) is a region of the brain located in the medial surface of the frontal lobe, and it plays an important role in the planning and execution of movements. In particular, the SMA is involved in the generation of movements that are guided by memory cues or internally generated plans, such as those involved in memory-guided movements.

Memory-guided movements are movements that are generated based on internal representations of the desired movement that are stored in memory. These representations may be based on previous experiences or motor plans that have been developed through practice or learning. The SMA is involved in the retrieval and selection of these internal representations and the generation of motor commands that control the movement.

Studies have shown that the SMA is particularly important for memory-guided movements that require temporal sequencing and coordination of multiple movements. For example, the SMA is involved in the generation of movements required to perform a *sequence* of motor tasks, such as playing a musical instrument or typing on a keyboard.

Overall, the SMA plays an important role in the generation of memory-guided movements by integrating information about the desired movement with information about the current state of the body and environment, and generating motor commands that control the movement. Dysfunction of the SMA can lead to deficits in the planning and execution of movements, highlighting the important role of this brain region in motor control.

The table shows the neural activities in relation to visual and memory guided movements

	M1	PM	SMA
Visual	+++++	+++	+
Memory	+++++	+	+++

The table depicts three motor areas in visually guided and memory-guided movement execution. The cells in the primary motor cortex (M1) fire equally well before either type of movement, visual or memory. The premotor cortex (PM) fires primarily in the visually guided task. The supplementary motor area (SMA) primarily fire in the internally guided task, memory.

An example is a test of bimanual movement. This two-dimensional task requires a correct movement sequence (Brinkman and Porter, 1983). The experiment is designed so the monkey will take the bait off a hole on a Perspex sheet. A normal monkey will use its preferred hand to push the bait from above and collect the falling bait with its non-preferred hand under the hole. However, a monkey with an SMA lesion lacks coordination between the two hands and cannot arrange correct movements to obtain the bait (Fig. 3.13).

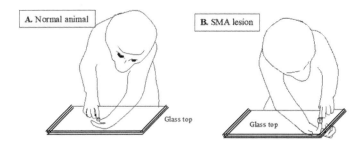

Figure 3.13. Monkey before and after SMA lesion. The figure above shows bimanual movement. The drawing at the top shows the monkey before the operation. The lower picture shows the monkey after the SMA lesion.

The monkey with an SMA lesion will not be able to perform simple memory-guided motor tasks after removing visual guidance. As described above, a monkey with an SMA lesion cannot carry out memory-guided movement. However, the monkey with an SMA lesion can perform some simple memory-guided movements with visual guidance. For example, a monkey is asked to raise its hand to reach for a peanut just above it. The monkey with an SMA lesion can perform this task using visually guided movement to compensate for the memory deficit. However, if the light is removed, the monkey with an SMA lesion will be unable to perform this simple task because the visually guided assistance is now abolished.

The test can examine the functional aspects of visual and memory-guided movements. For example, if we want to investigate the integrity of memory-guided movement, we can switch off the light to examine the consequences on the subject. After we turn off the light, the subject needs to use memory to guide the task. For example, the examiner asks the subject to walk to the door and open it. This test provides an estimation of the SMA function. If there is an SMA lesion, the subject will have difficulty performing a movement sequence when the light is off.

The table shows supplementary motor cortex and premotor cortex in response to visually and memory guided movement

	Visually guided movement		Memory guided movement
	Light on	Light off	Sequence
Lesion site SMA	+	0	0
PM	0	0	+

+: Movement is normal; 0: Movement is affected. SMA: supplementary motor cortex, PM: premotor cortex

Chapter 3: Cortex

Premovement Potential

Premovement potential can be recorded simultaneously from several scalp locations during self-paced voluntary extension movements (Fig. 3.14). For example, in right index finger movements, the subject was instructed to move the finger in their own time every five to ten seconds. EMG activity can be seen in the first trace. Before the onset of the EMG, a slowly rising wave can be seen in the EEG records. This is known as the *premovement potential*.

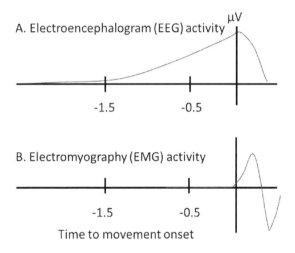

Figure 3.14. Schematic representation of the movement-related cortical potential. The above figure is a schematic representation of the movement-related cortical potential. The horizontal axis indicates the point of movement onset. The two line plots show the premovement potential of the brain and electromyography of the target muscles.

Neural bases of motor planning for Ready, Set, and Go

The neural bases for motor planning actions for the "ready, set, go" sequence involve the coordination of several brain regions, including the primary motor cortex (M1), the premotor cortex (PM), and the supplementary motor area (SMA).

Ready: During the "ready" phase, the motor cortex is involved in preparing the motor plan for the upcoming movement. This involves generating a plan for the movement and sending signals to the appropriate muscles to maintain a stable posture and prepare for the upcoming action. The neural basis for this phase involves the activation of the M1 and PM regions, which are involved in the initiation and preparation of movements, respectively.

Set: During the "set" phase, the motor cortex is involved in adjusting the motor plan and refining the movement strategy in response to feedback from sensory receptors. The neural basis for this phase involves the activation of the PM and SMA regions, which are involved in the selection and preparation of movements based on sensory feedback and task demands.

Go: During the "go" phase, the motor cortex is involved in activating specific muscle groups and coordinating their activity to generate the desired movement. The neural basis for this phase involves the activation of the M1 and SMA regions, which are involved in the execution and monitoring of movements in real-time.

Overall, the "ready, set, go" sequence involves the coordinated activity of several brain regions, including the M1, PM, and SMA, to generate and execute movements in a controlled and efficient manner. These regions work together to plan, prepare, and execute movements based on sensory feedback and task demands.

BRAIN INJURY

Brain injury can result in a variety of motor dysfunctions, depending on the location and extent of the injury. Motor dysfunction refers to the impairment or loss of motor function, including the ability to move, coordinate movements, and perform daily tasks.

Some common motor dysfunctions associated with brain injury include:

1. Paralysis: This is the complete loss of voluntary muscle control in one or more parts of the body. Paralysis can result from injury to the motor cortex, brainstem, or spinal cord.
2. Spasticity: This is the involuntary contraction of muscles, which can result in stiffness, tightness, and pain. Spasticity can result from injury to the corticospinal tract or damage to the motor neurons in the spinal cord.
3. Ataxia: This is the loss of coordination and balance, which can result in difficulty walking, standing, and performing other

movements. Ataxia can result from injury to the cerebellum, which is responsible for coordinating movements.
4. Tremors: This is the rhythmic shaking of one or more parts of the body. Tremors can result from injury to the basal ganglia, which are involved in the control of movement.
5. Apraxia: This is the inability to carry out voluntary movements, even though the muscles are intact and there is no paralysis. Apraxia can result from injury to the parietal cortex, which is involved in the planning and execution of movements.

Motor dysfunctions resulting from brain injury can have a significant impact on a person's ability to carry out daily activities and can affect their quality of life. Treatment for motor dysfunction may include physical therapy, occupational therapy, medications, and other interventions depending on the specific type and severity of the dysfunction.

Human motor dysfunction

Human motor dysfunction refers to any condition that impairs an individual's ability to control their movements. It can involve a wide range of problems, from minor difficulties with coordination to complete paralysis. Motor dysfunction can affect any part of the body, including the limbs, trunk, and face, and can be caused by a variety of factors, including genetic, developmental, and acquired conditions.

Chapter 3: Cortex

Some common types of human motor dysfunction include:

1. Traumatic Brain Injury: This is a type of acquired brain injury that can affect motor function, including balance, coordination, and movement control.
2. Movement Disorders: These conditions affect the speed, quality, and coordination of movements, resulting in tremors, rigidity, and/or involuntary movements. Examples include Parkinson's disease, Huntington's disease, and dystonia.
3. Cerebral Palsy: This is a group of neurological disorders that affect movement and coordination, caused by brain damage during development or shortly after birth.
4. Balance and Coordination Disorders: These disorders can make it difficult to maintain balance and coordinate movements, resulting in falls and difficulty with activities of daily living. Examples include ataxia and vertigo.
5. Stroke: A stroke occurs when blood flow to the brain is disrupted, resulting in brain damage and motor dysfunction.
6. Neuromuscular Disorders: These conditions affect the nerves, muscles, or both, causing muscle weakness, atrophy, and/or spasticity. Examples include muscular dystrophy, multiple sclerosis, and spinal muscular atrophy.
7. Orthopedic Injuries: These injuries can affect the joints, bones, and muscles, leading to pain, stiffness, and limited range of motion. Examples include sprains, strains, and fractures.

The causes of human motor dysfunction can be complex and multifaceted. They may include genetic mutations, brain injuries, infections, metabolic disorders, and exposure to toxins or drugs. Other factors that can contribute to motor dysfunction include stress, anxiety, and lifestyle factors like diet and exercise.

Treatment for human motor dysfunction depends on the underlying cause and the severity of the symptoms. Treatment may include medication, physical therapy, occupational therapy, speech therapy, and surgery. In some cases, assistive devices like braces or wheelchairs may be necessary to help individuals with motor dysfunction maintain their independence and mobility.

Brain Trauma

Brain trauma can result from various causes, such as car accidents, sports injuries, or crime-related events. Often, the symptoms of brain trauma are complex and present as a combination of motor, sensory, and cognitive dysfunction. Understanding the nature and extent of brain trauma is crucial in providing appropriate care and support for those affected.

Brain trauma can result in a wide range of motor dysfunctions depending on the location and severity of the injury. Motor dysfunctions can be broadly categorized into two types: primary motor dysfunction and secondary motor dysfunction.

Chapter 3: Cortex

Primary motor dysfunction results from direct damage to the brain's motor areas, such as the primary motor cortex, premotor cortex, basal ganglia, or cerebellum. This can cause weakness, paralysis, spasticity, tremors, or involuntary movements. The severity and extent of motor dysfunction can depend on the location and extent of the brain injury, as well as the individual's age, health, and previous motor function.

Secondary motor dysfunction results from damage to other areas of the brain that are not directly involved in motor control but play an important role in supporting motor function. For example, damage to the brain's sensory areas can impair proprioception or the sense of where the body is in space, affecting coordination and balance. In addition, damage to the frontal lobe can impair planning and decision-making, affecting the ability to initiate or execute motor movements.

Overall, the impact of brain trauma on motor function can be significant and can vary widely depending on the extent and location of the injury. However, with appropriate treatment and rehabilitation, many individuals can make significant improvements in motor function and quality of life.

Focal Brain Injury

Focal brain injury means the lesion is localized in a particular part of the brain. There are several types of focal brain injuries:

Cortical contusion

A cortical contusion is a type of brain injury that occurs when there is bruising or bleeding in the cerebral cortex. The cerebral cortex is responsible for many functions, including movement, sensation, perception, and consciousness.

Cortical contusions are most often caused by blunt force trauma to the head, such as in a car accident or a fall. The injury can also occur as a result of a direct blow to the head, such as in a sports-related injury or an assault.

Symptoms of a cortical contusion can vary depending on the severity and location of the injury. Some common symptoms may include headache, confusion, dizziness, nausea, vomiting, memory loss, seizures, and changes in vision, speech or movement. More severe contusions can cause coma, persistent unconsciousness, or even death.

Diffuse Brain Injury

Diffuse brain injury refers to a type of brain damage that affects multiple areas of the brain simultaneously, as opposed to a localized injury that affects a specific area. Diffuse brain injury is often caused by a blow to the head or a sudden acceleration or deceleration of the head, such as in a car accident; therefore, it is caused by a powerful impact such as shaking, rapid acceleration, and movement deceleration. The common symptoms of diffuse brain injury are spastic paralysis, cognitive deficits, disorientation, confusion, and behavioral depression. This type of injury can result in widespread damage to brain cells and the axons (nerve fibers) that connect them, leading to a range of neurological symptoms that can be difficult to predict and treat. Symptoms of a diffuse brain injury can include headache, confusion, memory problems, and changes in mood or behavior. In severe cases, diffuse brain injury can result in a persistent vegetative state or death.

Epidural haemorrhage

An epidural hemorrhage is a type of brain injury that occurs when there is bleeding between the skull and the outermost layer of the brain, called the dura mater (Fig. 3.15). A traumatic injury usually causes the bleeding in an epidural hemorrhage to the head, such as a fall, car accident, or assault. A common cause of an epidural hemorrhage is a lesion in the middle meningeal artery. Because the middle meningeal artery is relatively small, the symptoms develop gradually over several hours. An epidural hemorrhage can be life-threatening if not treated promptly and appropriately.

Motor dysfunction can occur as a result of an epidural hemorrhage, depending on the severity and location of the bleeding. The motor dysfunction may be temporary or permanent and can range from mild to severe.

Motor dysfunction resulting from an epidural hemorrhage may include weakness, paralysis, spasticity, abnormal movements, and changes in coordination and balance. The motor dysfunction may be limited to one side of the body or may affect both sides. In some cases, there may be associated sensory deficits, such as numbness or tingling in the affected limb.

The specific motor dysfunction associated with an epidural hemorrhage will depend on the location of the bleeding. For example, bleeding in the motor cortex, which is responsible for voluntary movement, can result in weakness or paralysis on one side of the body. Bleeding in the cerebellum, which is responsible for coordination and balance, can result in ataxia or uncoordinated movements.

Subdural hematoma

A subdural hematoma is a type of brain injury that occurs when there is bleeding between the dura mater and the arachnoid mater (Fig. 3.15). This bleeding can cause pressure to build up in the brain, leading to motor dysfunction, among other symptoms.

Chapter 3: Cortex

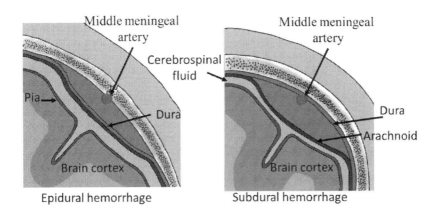

Figure 3.15. Epidural haemorrhage (left) and subdural haemorrhage (right).

This blood collection, or hematoma, can result from a head injury or trauma and can lead to pressure on the brain and brain damage. The symptoms develop rapidly and can be seen within a few hours. Subdural hematomas can range in severity from mild to life-threatening and treatment may involve surgery to remove the blood collection and relieve pressure on the brain.

Motor dysfunction resulting from a subdural hematoma can range from mild to severe, depending on the location and extent of the bleeding. The motor dysfunction may be temporary or permanent, and can include weakness, paralysis, spasticity, abnormal movements, and changes in coordination and balance. In some cases, there may also be associated sensory deficits, such as numbness or tingling in the affected limb.

The specific motor dysfunction associated with a subdural hematoma will depend on the location of the bleeding. For example, bleeding in the motor cortex, which is responsible for voluntary movement, can result in weakness or paralysis on one side of the body. Bleeding in the cerebellum, which is responsible for coordination and balance, can result in ataxia or uncoordinated movements.

Intracerebral hematoma

An intracerebral hematoma is bleeding inside the brain tissue. This is a type of brain injury in which blood accumulates within the brain tissue itself, usually as a result of a head injury or trauma. The buildup of blood can increase pressure within the skull and cause brain damage, leading to serious neurological symptoms such as weakness, seizures, and loss of consciousness.

Motor dysfunction resulting from an intracerebral hematoma can range from mild to severe, depending on the location and extent of the bleeding. The motor dysfunction may be temporary or permanent, and can include weakness, paralysis, spasticity, abnormal movements, and changes in coordination and balance. In some cases, there may also be associated sensory deficits, such as numbness or tingling in the affected limb.

The specific motor dysfunction associated with an intracerebral hematoma will depend on the location of the bleeding. For example, bleeding in the motor cortex, which is responsible for voluntary movement, can result in weakness or paralysis on one side of the body. Bleeding in the cerebellum, which is responsible for coordination and balance, can result in ataxia or uncoordinated movements.

Cerebellar Motor Syndrome

The cerebellar motor syndrome is a set of symptoms that occur due to damage to the cerebellum, a part of the brain responsible for coordinating movement and balance. The symptoms can include a range of motor dysfunction, including:

1. Ataxia: uncoordinated movements, such as stumbling or swaying when standing or walking
2. Dysmetria: difficulty judging the distance or force needed to complete a movement, leading to overreaching or underreaching
3. Dysdiadochokinesia: difficulty with rapid, alternating movements, such as tapping fingers or rapidly alternating foot movements
4. Intention tremor: tremors that occur when attempting to perform a movement, such as reaching for an object
5. Hypotonia: decreased muscle tone, leading to weakness and difficulty maintaining posture
6. In addition to these motor symptoms, cerebellar motor syndrome can also cause other neurological symptoms, such as

nystagmus (involuntary eye movements), vertigo, and slurred speech.

Cerebellar motor syndrome can be caused by a variety of factors, including stroke, trauma, infection, and degenerative diseases. Treatment will depend on the underlying cause of the syndrome and may include medications to manage symptoms, physical therapy to improve motor function, and occupational therapy to improve daily functioning. In some cases, surgery may be necessary to address the underlying cause of the cerebellar motor syndrome.

Cerebral Injury

A *cerebral injury* is common with a brain tumor or in a cerebrovascular accident:

Hemiparesis

Hemiparesis is a neurological condition characterized by weakness or partial paralysis of one side of the body (Fig. 3.16). It can affect any part of the body, including the arm, leg, and face, and can be caused by a variety of underlying conditions, such as stroke, brain injury, infection, tumor, or degenerative disease.

Chapter 3: Cortex

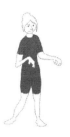

Figure 3.16. Hemiparesis

The severity of hemiparesis can vary widely, from mild weakness to complete paralysis, and the degree of impairment can depend on the location and extent of the underlying brain damage. Hemiparesis can also be accompanied by other neurological symptoms, such as numbness or tingling, difficulty with coordination or balance, and problems with speech or vision.

Treatment for hemiparesis typically involves a combination of physical therapy, occupational therapy, and medication, depending on the underlying cause and severity of the condition. Physical therapy may involve exercises to strengthen the affected muscles and improve range of motion, while occupational therapy may focus on activities of daily living, such as dressing, grooming, and eating.

Prognosis for hemiparesis can vary widely, depending on the cause and severity of the condition, but early and appropriate treatment can help improve outcomes and reduce the risk of complications.

Hemiplegia:

Hemiplegia is a type of motor dysfunction that results in the paralysis of one side of the body, including the arm, leg, and trunk. Hemiplegia is often caused by damage to the brain, such as a stroke or a traumatic brain injury.

The specific motor dysfunction associated with hemiplegia can vary depending on the location and extent of the brain damage. However, some common motor dysfunctions associated with hemiplegia include:

1. Weakness or complete paralysis of one side of the body: This is the most common motor dysfunction associated with hemiplegia.
2. Spasticity: This is the involuntary contraction of muscles, which can result in stiffness, tightness, and pain. Spasticity can affect the muscles on the affected side of the body in hemiplegia.
3. Abnormal movement patterns: Hemiplegia can result in abnormal movement patterns, such as a dragging foot or a bent knee, which can affect the ability to walk and perform other movements.
4. Poor coordination and balance: Hemiplegia can affect balance and coordination, making it difficult to perform activities such as standing, walking, and reaching.
5. Loss of fine motor skills: Hemiplegia can affect fine motor skills, making it difficult to perform activities that require precise hand movements, such as writing or using utensils.

Chapter 3: Cortex

Primary Motor Cortex Lesions

A primary motor cortex lesion refers to damage or injury to the primary motor cortex, which is the region of the brain that controls voluntary movement. This can result in motor deficits such as weakness, paralysis, or difficulty with movement coordination. Symptoms depend on the location and severity of the lesion. Treatment may involve rehabilitation and physical therapy to improve motor function. In some cases, surgery may be necessary to remove the lesion or alleviate pressure on the affected area of the brain.

Complete Destruction: Destruction of the primary motor cortex, or M1, can cause a loss of control of the distal muscles. The symptoms are paralysis of the hand, lower face, and foot. Because the distal muscles are involved in contralateral control, lesions on the motor cortex can cause muscle function loss on the opposite side.

Incomplete Destruction: Incomplete destruction of the primary motor cortex can cause paresis on the contralateral side of the body. The worst effects will be on the distal muscles, such as the finger muscles.

Spastic Dysarthria

Spastic dysarthria is a type of speech disorder that occurs due to damage to the upper motor neurons, which are responsible for controlling voluntary movements of the muscles used in speech.

This damage can be caused by a stroke, traumatic brain injury, or degenerative diseases like multiple sclerosis and amyotrophic lateral sclerosis (ALS).

Spastic dysarthria is characterized by slow, effortful speech with abnormal pauses between syllables, a strained or strangled voice quality, and limited range of motion in the jaw, tongue, and lips. This is because the upper motor neuron damage causes increased muscle tone or stiffness (spasticity) and decreased ability to control the muscles used in speech.

People with spastic dysarthria may also have difficulty with the rhythm and timing of speech, resulting in a monotone or robotic sounding voice. They may also have trouble with articulation, making it difficult to form certain sounds, especially those that require precise movements of the tongue and lips.

Treatment for spastic dysarthria may involve speech therapy to improve speech clarity, breathing techniques to enhance vocal support, and exercises to improve muscle tone and range of motion. In some cases, medications or surgery may be recommended to manage spasticity and improve speech function.

Cortex Abnormality

Cortex abnormality refers to any deviation from normal brain structure or function in the cortex, which is the outer layer of the brain responsible for cognitive and motor functions. Motor

Chapter 3: Cortex

dysfunction refers to a broad range of impairments in movement control and coordination.

Cortex lesions can be caused by a variety of factors, including:

1. Traumatic brain injury: A blow to the head can cause damage to the cortex and other brain structures, leading to a variety of motor and other neurological symptoms.
2. Stroke: A disruption of blood flow to the brain can cause damage to the cortex and other brain structures, leading to a variety of motor and other neurological symptoms.
3. Tumors: Cancerous or noncancerous growths can form in the cortex or other parts of the brain, leading to lesions and a variety of neurological symptoms.
4. Infections: Infections such as meningitis, encephalitis, or brain abscess can cause damage to the cortex and other brain structures, leading to a variety of neurological symptoms.
5. Autoimmune disorders: Certain autoimmune disorders, such as multiple sclerosis or lupus, can cause damage to the cortex and other brain structures, leading to a variety of neurological symptoms.
6. Neurodegenerative disorders: Disorders such as Alzheimer's disease, Huntington's disease, or Parkinson's disease can cause damage to the cortex and other brain structures over time, leading to a variety of neurological symptoms.

Common symptoms of cortical lesions may include:

1. Motor dysfunction: Lesions in the motor cortex can cause weakness, paralysis, and difficulty with coordination and movement. This can include difficulties with fine motor skills, such as writing or buttoning a shirt.
2. Sensory deficits: Lesions in the sensory cortex can cause sensory deficits, such as numbness, tingling, or loss of sensation in parts of the body.
3. Cognitive impairment: Lesions in areas of the cortex involved in cognitive function, such as the prefrontal cortex, can cause cognitive impairment, such as difficulty with attention, planning, decision-making, and memory.
4. Language difficulties: Lesions in the language areas of the cortex can cause language difficulties, such as difficulty with speaking, understanding language, or reading and writing.
5. Visual disturbances: Lesions in the visual cortex can cause visual disturbances, such as blindness, visual hallucinations, or other visual impairments.
6. Seizures: Some cortical lesions can cause seizures, which are sudden and uncontrollable electrical disturbances in the brain.

It is important to note that these symptoms can also be caused by other conditions, and the presence of one or more of these symptoms does not necessarily mean that a cortical lesion is present.

Apraxia

Apraxia is a neurological disorder characterized by the inability to perform a self-initiated or learned movement or sequence of movements. However, the subject understands the task and has intact motor output while there is a willingness to perform the movement. Apraxia can be seen in subjects with premotor or supplementary motor lesions. Subjects with apraxia may not be able to carry out a sequence of movements on request. Therefore, the desire and the capacity to move are present, but the person cannot execute the act.

Ideational Apraxia

Ideational apraxia is an abnormality in an overall ideational action plan. The subject cannot correctly order or sequence a series of movements to achieve a goal. Ideational apraxia can be seen in patients with SMA (supplementary motor cortex) lesions. Subjects cannot perform a sequence of movements, especially coordinated actions involving both hands. For example, they take a cigarette, light it, use an ashtray in the wrong order, display an inability to button up a shirt, or are unable to touch their nose. However, if self-initiation is not required, apraxia patients can perform those movements, such as scratching their nose if it itches.

Ideomotor Apraxia

This is a disorder at the interface between understanding and action of limb or facial movement. It relates to spatiotemporal errors in the positioning and orientation of the arm, hand, and fingers to the target and timing of the movements; however, the aim of the action is still unaffected.

- *Symptoms:* Ideomotor apraxia is the impaired ability to perform a skilled gesture with a limb upon verbal command. The deficit is typically identified with movements made to verbal command or imitation. It is a disorder characterized by deficits in properly performing communicative gestures (e.g., waving goodbye).
- Possible pathology: Disruptions of (1) the left parietal lobe, (2) the intrahemispheric association fibers, and (3) the dominant hemisphere motor association cortex
- Examples: Body part as object: Subjects substitute their fingers for the comb or toothbrush. If the subject is right-handed, it may indicate a left frontal abnormality.

Verbal apraxia or apraxia of speech

Difficulty with coordinating the movements needed for speech, resulting in difficulties with articulation and pronunciation.

Apraxia can be caused by a variety of factors, including stroke, traumatic brain injury, tumors, neurodegenerative disorders, and other neurological conditions. Treatment for apraxia involves rehabilitation, such as physical or occupational therapy, speech therapy, and other interventions aimed at improving motor planning, coordination, and overall function. The effectiveness of treatment depends on the severity and underlying cause of the condition.

Cortical Myoclonus

Cortical myoclonus is a symptom of a single muscle or group of muscle contractions that are very brief, involuntary, and random. They can be caused by neurological or metabolic disorders. There are two types of cortical myoclonus.

1) *Hypnic jerks:* Hypnic jerks present symptoms such as muscular twitching during sleep.

2) *Epilepsia partialis continua:* Epilepsia partialis continua presents symptoms such as unpredictable muscle twitching. These jerks can last for a few days.

Cerebellum

The cerebellum is a region of the brain located at the back of the skull, underneath the cerebral cortex. Although it only accounts for about 10% of the brain's total volume, the cerebellum is critical for the control and coordination of voluntary movements, posture, and balance.

The cerebellum receives information from various sensory systems, including the vestibular system (which senses changes in head position and movement), the visual system, and the somatosensory system (which provides information about touch, pressure, and position sense). It also receives input from the motor cortex and other regions of the brain involved in motor control.

Using this information, the cerebellum helps to fine-tune motor commands and adjust movement patterns in real time. It does this by comparing incoming sensory information with a "copy" of the motor command generated by the motor cortex. If there is a discrepancy between the intended movement and the actual movement, the cerebellum sends signals to the motor cortex to adjust the motor commands and improve the accuracy and precision of movement.

The cerebellum also plays a role in motor learning and adaptation. When we learn a new motor skill, such as riding a bike or playing an instrument, the cerebellum helps to consolidate the new information and refine the movement patterns. This allows us to perform the skill more smoothly and efficiently over time.

Damage or dysfunction of the cerebellum can lead to a range of motor deficits, including ataxia (loss of coordination and balance), dysmetria (difficulty with the accuracy and range of movement), and tremors. These deficits can have a significant impact on a person's ability to perform activities of daily living and may require rehabilitation and other forms of treatment.

Epilepsy

Epilepsy is a severe brain condition affecting more than seventy million people worldwide. Epilepsy incidence is at the highest risk in infants and older-age populations. Epilepsy is also called a *Jacksonian seizure*.

- Symptoms: The symptoms start with the twitching of a small group of muscles in one part of the body (hands, feet, or corner of the mouth). Then, the twitching spreads and becomes a full tonic-clonic convulsion of the whole body. It is a condition of recurrent and unprovoked seizures.
- Pathology: The concept is a distortion of excitation and inhibition in the brain. Seizures start from repeated discharges from groups of neurons, which arise from excessive excitation or loss of inhibition. An EEG may show that local excitatory cortical activity (temporal lobe) spreads to adjacent areas.

CHAPTER 4: BASAL GANGLIA AND MOVEMENT QUALITY

The basal ganglia are a group of interconnected subcortical structures located deep within the brain that play a critical role in the control of movement. They receive input from several brain regions, including the cortex, thalamus, and brainstem, and send output to motor regions of the brain, including the primary motor cortex (M1).

The basal ganglia are involved in a range of motor functions, including the selection, initiation, and control of movements. They work together with other motor regions of the brain, such as the cerebellum and motor cortex, to regulate movement quality and ensure that movements are performed smoothly and efficiently.

The basal ganglia facilitate voluntary movements and inhibit competing movements that could interfere with the desired movement. They help initiate and smooth out muscle movements, suppress involuntary movements, and coordinate changes in posture.

Chapter 4: Basal Ganglia and Movement Quality

Disruptions in the basal ganglia can lead to movement disorders, such as Parkinson's disease, Huntington's disease, and dystonia. These disorders are characterized by impairments in movement quality, including tremors, rigidity, and bradykinesia (slowness of movement).

A person with a basal ganglia lesion may have difficulties starting, stopping, or sustaining movement. For example, the patient could have difficulty controlling speech, movement, and posture.

Overall, the basal ganglia play a critical role in regulating movement quality and ensuring that movements are performed smoothly and efficiently. Dysfunction in the basal ganglia can lead to a range of motor deficits and movement disorders, highlighting the importance of these structures in motor control.

STRUCTURE AND FUNCTION

Anatomy

The basal ganglia consist of a group of brain subcortical nuclei located at the base of the forebrain and top of the midbrain (Fig. 4.1). The main components of basal ganglia are the striatum, globus pallidus, substantia nigra, and subthalamic nucleus, which form the basal ganglia motor circuits.

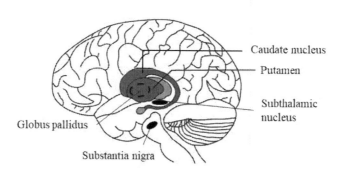

Figure 4.1. Basal ganglia. This figure shows a lateral view of the brain. It shows the components of the basal ganglia, including the caudate, putamen, globus pallidus, subthalamic nucleus, and substantial nigra.

- *Striatum:* The striatum consists of the *dorsal striatum* (caudate nucleus and putamen) and the *ventral striatum* (nucleus accumbens and olfactory tubercle) (Fig. 4.2). It is for motor learning, memory, rhythm, and movement stability.
- *Globus pallidus:* The globus pallidus (GP) consists of the external (GPe) and internal (GPi) parts. The globus pallidus maintains stability and keeps accurate timing of voluntary movements.
- *Substantia nigra:* The substantia nigra lies in the midbrain. Human substantia nigra neurons contain melanin. Substantia nigra can be divided into pars compacta (dorsal) and pars reticulata. The substantia nigra executes a movement already underway. It can influence the direct and indirect pathways of

Chapter 4: Basal Ganglia and Movement Quality

basal ganglia motor circuitry to activate and adjust the frequency of the movements. The substantia nigra helps to modulate movements via the neurotransmitter dopamine. It is involved in the disinhibition of basal ganglia output. It does not initiate action but executes it when it is already underway.

- *Subthalamic nucleus:* Located in the rostral part of the midbrain dorsal to the cerebral peduncle, the subthalamic nucleus activates the final output of basal ganglia.

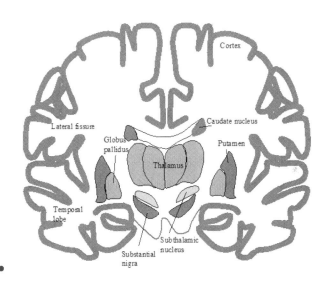

Figure 4.2. Coronal section of the brain. This figure is from a coronal section of the brain through the hypothalamus. It shows the locations of the basal ganglia, including the striatum (caudate and putamen), globus pallidus, subthalamic nucleus, and substantia nigra.

Function

Generally speaking, the basal ganglia ensure the quality of voluntary movement by selecting or inhibiting specific motor synergies. It regulates the quality of actions, including stability and automatic prediction. Furthermore, basal ganglia arrange the sequencing of automated activities.

Putamen and motor control

The putamen

is a key brain structure located within the basal ganglia, which is a collection of nuclei involved in various aspects of motor control.

The striatum coordinates several aspects of cognition, including movement planning, decision-making, motivation, reinforcement, and reward perception. The putamen is particularly important in the regulation of voluntary movements, including the selection, initiation, and execution of movements.

One way the putamen contributes to motor control is by receiving and integrating sensory information from the cerebral cortex, which is involved in higher cognitive functions such as perception, attention, and decision-making. This sensory information is then processed and transmitted to other regions of the basal ganglia, such as the globus pallidus, substantia nigra, and thalamus, which are involved in the regulation of motor activity.

Chapter 4: Basal Ganglia and Movement Quality

The putamen is also involved in motor learning, which is the process of acquiring new motor skills or improving existing ones through practice and repetition. Research has shown that the putamen is particularly active during the early stages of motor learning. Its activity decreases as the skill becomes more automatic and requires less conscious effort.

Dysfunction of the putamen has been associated with various movement disorders, including Parkinson's disease, Huntington's disease, and dystonia, which are characterized by abnormal movements or postures. For example, in Parkinson's disease, the degeneration of dopamine-producing neurons in the substantia nigra results in decreased dopamine levels in the putamen, leading to motor symptoms such as tremors, rigidity, and bradykinesia (slowness of movement).

In summary, the putamen plays a critical role in motor control by integrating sensory information and regulating the selection, initiation, and execution of voluntary movements. The putamen is also involved in motor learning, and dysfunction of the putamen can result in various movement disorders.

Globus pallidus and motor control

The globus pallidus is a structure located within the basal ganglia, a collection of nuclei in the brain that are involved in the regulation of motor control. The globus pallidus is divided into two subregions, the external segment (GPe) and the internal segment (GPi), which have distinct functions in motor control.

The GPe receives input from the striatum, which includes the caudate and putamen, and sends inhibitory signals to the subthalamic nucleus (STN). The GPi, in turn, receives inhibitory signals from the GPe and sends output to the thalamus, which relays information to the motor cortex. The net effect of this circuitry is to regulate the activity of the thalamus and motor cortex, thereby influencing motor behavior.

The globus pallidus is involved in a variety of motor functions, including the selection and initiation of voluntary movements, as well as the suppression of unwanted movements. In Parkinson's disease, a neurodegenerative disorder that affects motor function, the degeneration of dopaminergic neurons in the substantia nigra leads to decreased dopamine levels in the striatum, which can result in increased activity in the GPe and decreased activity in the GPi. This shift in activity can lead to the characteristic motor symptoms of Parkinson's disease, including tremors, rigidity, and bradykinesia (slowness of movement).

Deep brain stimulation (DBS), a surgical treatment for movement disorders, can be used to target the globus pallidus. In Parkinson's disease, DBS can be used to stimulate the GPi, which can alleviate the motor symptoms associated with the disease. DBS of the GPe can also be used to treat dystonia, a movement disorder characterized by sustained muscle contractions that cause twisting and repetitive movements or abnormal postures.

Lesion to the external globus pallidus causes hypokinesia. Conversely, blocking input to the external globus pallidus causes hyperkinesia. For example, injecting a GABA blocker (bicuculline) into the external globus pallidus causes hyperkinesia. This is due to blocking the striatal GABA inhibition input.

Lesions on the internal globus pallidus cause hyperkinesia. Animal study shows that blocking the internal globus pallidus reduces the frequency and slows the movement's speed.

In summary, the globus pallidus plays an important role in motor control by regulating the activity of the thalamus and motor cortex. Dysfunction of the globus pallidus can result in various movement disorders, and DBS can be used to target this structure to alleviate symptoms.

Example

The globus pallidus is involved in the control of stability of movement. This was demonstrated by a cooling experiment where a monkey was trained to do an elbow joint extension following a visual instruction.

Experiment design: An electronic cooling device was surgically implanted into the globus pallidus of the monkey. This device could be remotely controlled to alter the temperature of the globus pallidus. Results:

1. The results showed that when the temperature of the globus pallidus was lowered, the quality of elbow joint extension movement was affected. EMG activity recorded from the triceps and biceps showed that the cooling affected the quality of movement in terms of speed, size, and starting and finishing time points.
2. Speed, magnitude, initiation, completion, and rebound: After the temperature of the globus pallidus was lowered, the elbow extension movement showed the following: 1) The movement was slower than required; 2) The degree of movement was smaller than needed; 3) The starting point for the movement was later; 4) The finishing point of the movement was earlier than required; and 5) The elbow extension movement can rebound back toward the original position shortly after starting. Therefore, lesions on the globus pallidus can cause movement to become unstable (small, slow, or not starting correctly).

Chapter 4: Basal Ganglia and Movement Quality

3. Sequential movements: Globus pallidus neurons are involved in learning repetitive sequential movements. A study showed that a monkey was asked to perform a repetitive and proper sequential action this time. It had to perform a sequential movement consisting of wrist flexion toward a target, hold it for one second, and then return to the starting point. The results showed that the globus pallidus neurons had a minimal response in the first trial. However, in the subsequent trials, the discharge of globus pallidus neurons increased following multiple repetitions of the movement. More importantly, there was an additional burst of neural activity. This activity of globus pallidus neurons is seen as a predictive activity for repetitive movements. However, this particular burst did not exist in the monkey who performed randomized movements, which were unpredictable.

Subthalamic nucleus and motor control

The subthalamic nucleus (STN) is a small, lens-shaped structure located deep within the brain, specifically within the basal ganglia, a group of nuclei involved in motor control. The STN is known to play a crucial role in regulating movement, particularly through its connections with the primary motor cortex and other brain regions involved in movement control.

The STN receives input from the cortex, striatum, and other basal ganglia structures and sends output to the globus pallidus interna

(GPi) and substantia nigra pars reticulata (SNr), which in turn modulate the thalamus and ultimately control movement. The STN is believed to act as a "brake" on movement, inhibiting unwanted movements and facilitating the execution of desired movements.

Lesions on the substantia nigra lead to a reduced frequency of movement. Furthermore, they slow down the speed of that movement.

Deep brain stimulation (DBS) of the STN has been used as a therapeutic approach for Parkinson's disease and other movement disorders. The stimulation of the STN can improve motor symptoms, such as tremors, rigidity, and bradykinesia, by increasing the activity of the GPi and SNr and restoring the balance between excitatory and inhibitory signals in the basal ganglia.

In summary, the subthalamic nucleus is a key component of the basal ganglia network and plays a critical role in the regulation of motor control. Dysfunction of the STN can lead to movement disorders, and DBS of the STN can be used as a therapeutic approach to improve motor symptoms in certain conditions.

Substantia nigra and motor control

The substantia nigra (SN) lies in the midbrain and plays a vital role in motor control. The SN contains two distinct regions, the substantia nigra pars compacta (SNc), and substantia nigra pars reticulata (SNr).

Chapter 4: Basal Ganglia and Movement Quality

The SNc contains dopaminergic neurons that project to the striatum and play a critical role in the modulation of motor activity. The SNr plays a critical role in inhibiting unwanted movements and facilitating desired movements, similar to the STN. Loss of dopaminergic neurons in the SNc is a hallmark of Parkinson's disease and is responsible for the motor symptoms associated with the disorder, such as tremors, rigidity, and bradykinesia.

Lesions on the subthalamic nucleus cause hyperkinesia.

Therefore, the SN is an essential structure for motor control, and its dysfunction can lead to movement disorders. Parkinson's disease is a classic example of an illness that results from the degeneration of dopaminergic neurons in the SNc. Treatments for Parkinson's disease, such as dopamine replacement therapy and deep brain stimulation, target the SN to restore proper motor function.

Summary of the mechanism of action: Basal ganglia inhibit "automatic" postural activity that provides the basis for allowing voluntary movement; therefore, it prevents unwanted muscle activity during focal tasks. Basal ganglia can regulate several different types of movement simultaneously (not single activities). The final output of the basal ganglia is the disinhibition that allows movement. Usually, there is a constant inhibitory activity in the internal globus pallidus.

The basal ganglia motor loop

The basal ganglia motor loop is a circuit within the basal ganglia that is responsible for the control of movement. The loop consists of several nuclei, including the striatum, globus pallidus, subthalamic nucleus, and substantia nigra.

The basal ganglia motor loop is organized in a series of parallel pathways that process information from the cortex and modulate motor activity. The loop receives input from the cortex, which projects to the striatum. The striatum consists of two main regions, the caudate nucleus and the putamen, which process different types of information. The caudate nucleus receives input from the prefrontal cortex and is involved in cognitive functions, while the putamen receives input from the motor and sensory cortex and is involved in motor functions.

The output of the striatum is modulated by the globus pallidus interna (GPi) and substantia nigra pars reticulata (SNr), which inhibit the thalamus and ultimately modulate cortical activity. The GPi and SNr receive input from the striatum through two parallel pathways, the direct and indirect pathways.

The direct pathway facilitates movement by disinhibiting the thalamus, while the indirect pathway inhibits movement by increasing the inhibition of the thalamus. The subthalamic nucleus (STN) acts as a switch that modulates the activity of the direct and indirect pathways. The STN receives input from the cortex and projects to the GPi/SNr, modulating their activity.

Chapter 4: Basal Ganglia and Movement Quality

Dysfunction of the basal ganglia motor loop can lead to movement disorders such as Parkinson's and Huntington's diseases. Therefore, understanding the circuitry of the basal ganglia motor loop is essential for developing treatments for these disorders.

PATHWAYS

Basal Ganglia Motor Regulatory Pathways

The following figure shows the regulatory pathways of motor control in the basal ganglia of a healthy person.

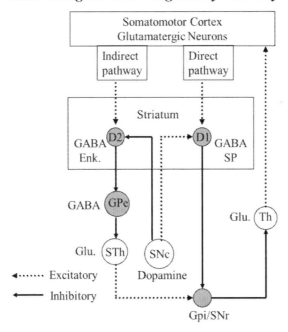

Basal Ganglia Motor Regulatory Pathways

Figure 4.3. The regulatory pathways of motor control in the basal ganglia of a healthy person. The figure shows a balance of direct, indirect, and dopaminergic pathways that regulate basal ganglia output. The lines represent the output of the direct and indirect pathways. The dotted arrow represents the excitatory subthalamopallidal pathway (horizontal white connection), which is under the inhibitory control of the external globus pallidus. The thickness of the connection lines indicates the relative contribution of each pathway. Abbreviations: D1 and D2: dopamine D1 and D2 receptors; GABA: gamma-aminobutyric acid; Enk, enkephalin; SP, substance P; GPe, globus pallidus external; STh, subthalamic nucleus; SNc, substantial nigra compacta; GPi, globus pallidus internal; Glu, glutamate; Th, thalamus

Direct pathway: The direct pathway is also called the excitatory pathway (fig. 22). Glutamatergic neurons (M1, PM, and SMA) project to the dendritic spine of the striatum's medium spiny neurons (GABAergic neurons). The striatal GABAergic neurons are co-localized with substance P and dynorphin and project to the internal globus pallidus and substantia nigra (GPi/SNr, GABAergic neurons). These neurons project to the thalamus (glutamatergic neurons) and excite the cortex (M1, PM, and SMA).

Indirect pathway: The indirect pathway is also called the *inhibitory pathway*. Glutamatergic neurons from the cortex (M1, PM, and SMA) project to striatal medium spiny neurons, which are GABAergic neurons co-localized with enkephalin and neurotensin. Striatal medium spiny neurons project to the neuron part (GABAergic neurons) of the external globus pallidus. These neurons then project to the glutamatergic neurons of the subthalamic nucleus (STN). The STN neurons then project to the internal globus pallidus and substantia nigra reticulata (GABAergic neurons) and then to the thalamus (glutamatergic neurons), which excite the motor cortex (M1, PM, and SMA).

Terminologies used in describing basal ganglia motor dysfunction

Hypokinesia or akinesia: the person lacks spontaneous movement.

Involuntary movement: an automatic movement that is abnormal to skeletal muscles.

Hyperkinesia: an excess of activities seen in Huntington's chorea and dystonia.

Bradykinesia: the slowness of movement.

Differences between basal ganglia motor syndrome and extrapyramidal syndrome

Basal ganglia motor syndrome and extrapyramidal syndrome are related terms that describe movement disorders caused by dysfunction of the basal ganglia and other structures that modulate movement.

The term "extrapyramidal syndrome" refers to a broad category of movement disorders that are caused by dysfunction of the extrapyramidal system, which includes the basal ganglia, as well as other structures such as the substantia nigra and the thalamus. An extrapyramidal syndrome features a range of motor dysfunctions, including tremors, rigidity, bradykinesia, and postural instability.

Basal ganglia motor syndrome is a specific type of extrapyramidal syndrome caused by dysfunction of the basal ganglia motor loop, a circuit within the basal ganglia responsible for the control of movement. Basal ganglia motor syndrome includes movement disorders such as Parkinson's disease, Huntington's disease, dystonia, and Tourette's syndrome.

In summary, extrapyramidal syndrome is a broad term that refers to movement disorders caused by dysfunction of the extrapyramidal system. In contrast, basal ganglia motor syndrome is a specific type of extrapyramidal syndrome caused by dysfunction of the basal ganglia motor loop. Both terms describe movement disorders resulting from dysfunction of similar neural circuits, but basal ganglia motor syndrome is a more specific and well-defined term.

ABNORMALITIES

Movement quality alterations

Chapter 4: Basal Ganglia and Movement Quality

Movement frequency changes

A variety of factors, including neurological disorders, medications, and physiological changes, can cause changes in movement frequency.

1. Neurological disorders: Certain neurological disorders, such as Parkinson's disease, Huntington's disease, and Tourette's syndrome, can cause changes in movement frequency. For example, Parkinson's disease is characterized by bradykinesia, or slowness of movement, while rapid, involuntary movements characterize Tourette's syndrome.
2. Medications: Certain medications, such as antipsychotics and antidepressants, can cause changes in movement frequency as a side effect. For example, some antipsychotics can cause akathisia, a condition characterized by restless movements and an inability to sit still.
3. Physiological changes: Changes in physiological factors, such as fatigue or stress, can also affect movement frequency. For example, fatigue can cause slowness of movement and decreased frequency, while stress can cause increased movement frequency.
4. Environmental factors: Changes in environmental factors, such as temperature or humidity, can also affect movement frequency. For example, cold temperatures can cause decreased movement frequency, while warm temperatures can cause increased movement frequency.

Overall, changes in movement frequency can be caused by a variety of factors, and a thorough medical evaluation is necessary to determine the underlying cause. Treatment may involve medications, physical therapy, and lifestyle modifications to manage the underlying condition and improve movement frequency.

Hyperkinesia

Hyperkinesia is a term used to describe excessive, involuntary movements that are often rapid and jerky in nature. It is a type of movement disorder that can be caused by a variety of underlying neurological conditions or medications.

There are several different types of hyperkinesia, including:

1. Chorea: Rapid, involuntary movements that can affect any part of the body, including the face, arms, and legs. Chorea is often seen in conditions such as Huntington's disease and Sydenham's chorea.
2. Dystonia: Involuntary muscle contractions that cause twisting and repetitive movements or abnormal postures. Dystonia can affect one or more body parts and may be caused by a variety of underlying conditions, including cerebral palsy and Parkinson's disease.
3. Myoclonus: Sudden, brief muscle contractions or jerks that can affect any part of the body. Myoclonus can be caused by a

variety of underlying conditions, including epilepsy and metabolic disorders.

4. Tics: Repetitive, involuntary movements or vocalizations that can be simple or complex in nature. Tics are often seen in conditions such as Tourette's syndrome.

Hyperkinesia can have a significant impact on an individual's quality of life, affecting their ability to perform daily activities and participate in social interactions.

Tremor

Tremor is an involuntary, rhythmic movement or shaking of a body part. It can affect any part of the body, but most commonly occurs in the hands, arms, head, face, vocal cords, and trunk. Tremors can be mild or severe, and can range from barely noticeable to so severe that they interfere with daily activities.

Tremors can be caused by a variety of factors, including neurological disorders, such as Parkinson's disease or essential tremor, as well as other medical conditions, medications, or substance abuse. In some cases, tremors may be caused by emotional stress, fatigue, or caffeine intake.

The type of tremor a person experiences can also vary. Some of the common types of tremors include:

1. Resting tremor: A tremor that occurs when the body part is at rest, and decreases or disappears with movement.

2. Postural tremor: A tremor that occurs when the body part is held against gravity, such as holding a cup or a phone.
3. Kinetic tremor: A tremor that occurs during voluntary movement, such as reaching for an object.
4. Intention tremor: A tremor that occurs during precise movements, such as touching the nose or finger-to-nose test.

The treatment of tremors depends on the underlying cause and severity of the condition. Some treatments may include medications, physical therapy, or deep brain stimulation. Additionally, lifestyle modifications such as relaxation techniques, stress management, and avoiding triggers may also be recommended to help manage tremors

Rapid Irregular Jerks

Rapid irregular jerks refer to sudden, involuntary movements that are typically brief and unpredictable in their timing and direction. These movements can affect various parts of the body, including the limbs, head, face, and torso, and may occur in isolation or in clusters.

Rapid irregular jerks can be a symptom of several different neurological conditions, including:

1. Myoclonus: A neurological condition characterized by sudden, brief muscle contractions that can occur spontaneously or in

response to a stimulus, such as a loud noise or sudden movement.
2. Choreiform movements: A type of involuntary movement characterized by rapid, irregular, and jerky movements that can affect the limbs, face, and trunk. Choreiform movements are a hallmark symptom of Huntington's disease.
3. Dystonia: A neurological condition characterized by involuntary muscle contractions that can cause twisting, repetitive movements or abnormal postures.
4. Tardive dyskinesia: A movement disorder that can be caused by long-term use of certain medications, characterized by rapid, irregular movements of the face and limbs.
5. Tourette's syndrome: A neurological condition characterized by involuntary tics, including sudden, rapid jerks of the limbs or other body parts.

Tardive Dyskinesia

Tardive dyskinesia (TD) is a neurological disorder characterized by involuntary and repetitive movements of the face, tongue, mouth, and other body parts. These movements can include grimacing, puckering of the lips, tongue protrusion, blinking, and rapid eye movements. The movements may be rapid, jerky, and unpredictable in their timing and direction. In some cases, TD can also affect the limbs and trunk.

TD can develop as a side effect of long-term use of certain medications, particularly antipsychotic medications used to treat psychiatric conditions such as schizophrenia, bipolar disorder, and depression.

The exact cause of TD is not fully understood, but it is thought to be related to changes in dopamine receptors in the brain, which can be affected by long-term use of certain medications.

Risk factors for developing TD include older age, female, higher doses of medication, and longer duration of treatment. The risk of developing TD increases with longer duration of treatment and higher doses of medications.

Hypokinesia

Hypokinesia is a term used to describe a reduction in voluntary movements, resulting in slowed or decreased physical activity. It is a type of movement disorder that can be caused by a variety of underlying neurological conditions or medications.

There are several different types of hypokinesia, including:

1. Bradykinesia: Slowness of voluntary movements, often seen in conditions such as Parkinson's disease.
2. Akinesia: Inability to initiate voluntary movements, often seen in advanced Parkinson's disease.
3. Rigidity: Stiffness or resistance to movement, often seen in conditions such as Parkinson's disease or dystonia.
4. Catatonia: A state of unresponsiveness, decreased activity, and abnormal postures, often seen in certain psychiatric disorders.

Hypokinesia can significantly impact an individual's quality of life, affecting their ability to perform daily activities and participate in social interactions. Treatment may involve medications like levodopa or dopamine agonists or other therapies, such as deep brain stimulation or physical therapy. Rehabilitation programs may be recommended to help improve motor control, increase physical activity, and reduce the severity of hypokinetic symptoms.

Akathisia

Akathisia is a movement disorder characterized by a feeling of inner restlessness and a compelling need to move. It can be a side effect of certain medications, particularly antipsychotics and antidepressants. Akathisia may also occur as a symptom of certain medical conditions, such as Parkinson's disease, or as a result of drug withdrawal.

The symptoms of akathisia can include: A feeling of restlessness or agitation; A compulsive need to move; Pacing or rocking back and forth; Inability to sit still; Fidgeting or tapping of feet; Tremors or muscle stiffness

Akathisia can be distressing and can interfere with daily activities, sleep, and overall quality of life.

Muscle tone changes

Muscle tone changes can be caused by a variety of factors, including neurological disorders, medications, and physical injury or trauma.

1. Neurological disorders: Certain neurological disorders, such as Parkinson's disease, Huntington's disease, and cerebral palsy, can cause changes in muscle tone. For example, Parkinson's disease is characterized by muscle rigidity, or increased muscle tone, while cerebral palsy is characterized by spasticity, or increased muscle tone and stiffness.
2. Medications: Certain medications, such as muscle relaxants and sedatives, can cause changes in muscle tone as a side effect. For example, muscle relaxants can cause decreased muscle tone, while sedatives can cause increased muscle tone.
3. Physical injury or trauma: Physical injury or trauma, such as a spinal cord injury or stroke, can cause changes in muscle tone.

For example, spinal cord injury can cause spasticity, or increased muscle tone, while stroke can cause flaccidity or decreased muscle tone.

4. Other factors: Other factors that can affect muscle tone include stress, fatigue, and dehydration. Stress and fatigue can cause muscle stiffness and increased muscle tone, while dehydration can cause decreased muscle tone.

Treatment may involve medications, physical therapy, and lifestyle modifications to manage the underlying condition and improve muscle tone.

Posture abnormality

Motor control alterations can contribute to posture abnormalities by disrupting the alignment and distribution of weight through the body. Poor motor control can lead to muscle imbalances, decreased range of motion, and inefficient movement patterns, which can contribute to the development of postural abnormalities.

For example, muscle weakness or spasticity can lead to an imbalance in muscle tension, leading to a forward head or slouched posture. In addition, changes in muscle tone, such as increased or decreased muscle stiffness, can affect joint mobility and contribute to postural abnormalities.

Motor control alterations can also result from neurological conditions, such as Parkinson's disease, which can cause tremors, rigidity, and bradykinesia (slowness of movement). These symptoms can affect posture and balance, leading to an increased risk of falls and other injuries.

Physical therapy can help improve motor control by addressing underlying neurological and musculoskeletal issues, such as weakness, spasticity, and tremors. Treatment may involve a combination of exercises to improve strength and flexibility, as well as balance and coordination training. In addition, assistive devices, such as braces or orthotics, may be used to support proper alignment and reduce the risk of falls.

Improving motor control can also help prevent the development of postural abnormalities or slow their progression, improving overall movement efficiency and quality of life.

Extrapyramidal Syndrome

Extrapyramidal syndrome (EPS) is a group of movement disorders that can occur as a side effect of certain medications, particularly antipsychotic medications. These disorders affect the motor system and can cause a range of symptoms, including muscle stiffness, tremors, slow movements, and difficulty with balance and coordination.

The term "extrapyramidal" refers to the part of the nervous system that controls movement and is not part of the pyramidal tract, which is responsible for voluntary motor control. EPS is thought to be caused by an imbalance of dopamine, a neurotransmitter that plays a key role in regulating movement, in the brain.

There are several types of EPS, including dystonia, akathisia, parkinsonism, and tardive dyskinesia. Dystonia causes involuntary muscle contractions that can cause repetitive movements, while akathisia causes restlessness and a feeling of inner discomfort. Parkinsonism causes symptoms similar to Parkinson's disease, such as tremors, rigidity, and slowness of movement. Tardive dyskinesia is a severe form of EPS that can occur after prolonged use of antipsychotic medications and is characterized by involuntary, repetitive movements of the face, tongue, and limbs.

Treatment of EPS depends on the specific symptoms and their severity, and may include adjusting the dosage or type of medication, adding another medication to counteract EPS symptoms, or discontinuing the antipsychotic medication altogether. In some cases, additional medications such as benzodiazepines or anticholinergic agents may be prescribed to help manage EPS symptoms.

Physical therapy for motor dysfunction

Physical therapy can be an effective treatment option for various types of motor dysfunction, which refer to any impairment or difficulty in movement. Motor dysfunction can be caused by a variety of factors, including neurological disorders, musculoskeletal injuries, and age-related changes.

Physical therapists can help patients with motor dysfunction by creating individualized treatment plans that focus on improving their mobility, strength, balance, and coordination. Depending on the specific condition and its severity, physical therapy may involve a range of interventions, including:

1. Exercises: Physical therapists use exercises to improve strength, flexibility, and range of motion. These exercises can be customized for each patient based on their specific needs.
2. Gait training: Gait training is a type of exercise that focuses on improving walking and balance. Physical therapists use various techniques to help patients walk more efficiently and safely.
3. Manual therapy: Manual therapy techniques, such as massage and joint mobilization, can relieve pain and stiffness and improve mobility.
4. Neuromuscular re-education: Neuromuscular re-education involves helping patients regain control of their movements by teaching them how to move in a more coordinated and efficient way.
5. Assistive devices: Physical therapists may recommend assistive devices, such as braces or crutches, to support mobility and prevent falls.

Physical therapy can also help manage motor dysfunction caused by neurological disorders like Parkinson's disease and stroke. For example, physical therapy can help Parkinson's disease patients improve their gait and balance, reduce muscle stiffness, and increase their overall activity level. Physical therapy can also help stroke patients regain strength and coordination in the affected limbs, improve their ability to perform daily activities, and prevent complications such as muscle contractures.

Therefore, physical therapy is an important treatment option for motor dysfunction and can help patients achieve greater mobility, independence, and overall quality of life. A physical therapist will conduct an initial evaluation of the patient, create an individualized treatment plan, and monitor progress over time. Physical therapy may be provided in various settings, including hospitals, clinics, schools, and rehabilitation centers, as well as in the patient's home.

Deep brain stimulation

Deep brain stimulation (DBS) is a treatment option that can be used to help manage motor control disorders, such as Parkinson's disease, essential tremor, and dystonia. In these conditions, the brain's motor circuits are affected, resulting in involuntary movements, tremors, and other motor symptoms.

DBS involves implanting a small electrode in the brain, which is connected to a pulse generator (battery) implanted under the skin in the chest or abdomen. The electrode delivers electrical impulses to specific areas of the brain involved in motor control, which can help regulate abnormal brain activity and improve motor symptoms.

Studies have shown that DBS can significantly improve motor symptoms in people with Parkinson's disease, essential tremor, and dystonia, and may allow for reduced medication use and improved quality of life. DBS can also help manage symptoms in people with other movement disorders, such as Huntington's disease, Tourette's syndrome, and tardive dyskinesia.

DBS is typically reserved for people who have not responded well to other treatments for their motor control disorder, such as medications, physical therapy, or lifestyle modifications. As with any surgical procedure, DBS carries some risks and potential side effects, including infection, bleeding, and neurological complications.

DBS is not a cure for motor control disorders, but it can be an effective treatment option for managing symptoms and improving quality of life for some people. It is important to discuss the potential benefits and risks of DBS with a healthcare professional to determine if it is an appropriate treatment option.

Parkinson's Disease

Parkinson's disease is a motor dysfunction caused by basal ganglia lesions. Usually, it affects older adults over forty-five years of age. The disease features are akinesia, tremors, and muscular rigidity.

For example, patients can have a mask-like facial expression, a shuffling gait, a droopy posture, and a rhythmical muscular tremor.

Parkinson's disease is a neurodegenerative disorder that affects movement. It is caused by the progressive degeneration of dopamine-producing neurons in the brain, leading to a shortage of dopamine and subsequent motor dysfunction (Fig. 4.4).

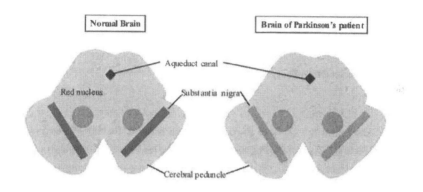

Figure 4.4. Sections of the midbrain, normal brain (left) and brain of Parkinson's patient (right). The figure shows two sections of the midbrain. The image on the left shows the normal substantia nigra. The image on the right shows the substantia nigra from a Parkinson's patient. Pigmented neurons were lost from the substantia nigra, giving an abnormally pale appearance. In Parkinson's disease, the neurons that usually contain melanin are now occupied by Lewy bodies inside the neurons as a spherical inclusion body.

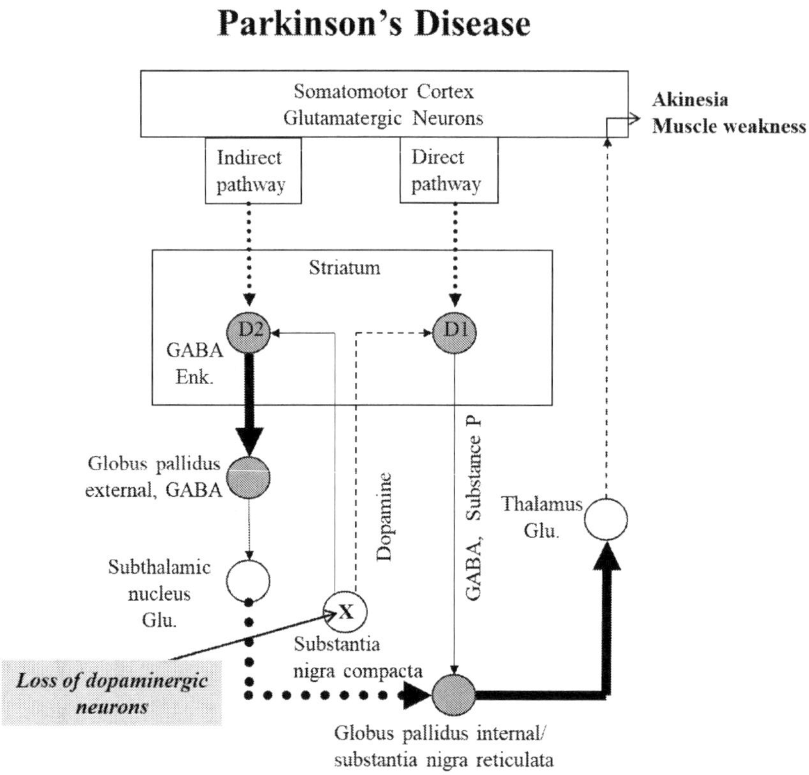

Parkinson's Disease

Figure 4.5. Parkinson's disease has altered direct and indirect pathway signals. The figure shows that Parkinson's disease loses dopaminergic neurons in the substantia nigra compacta leading to reduced projection to the striatum. In the direct pathway, there is a decreased output to the globus pallidus internal via the D1 receptor. In the indirect pathway, there is an increased output to the globus pallidus internal via the D2 receptor.

The motor symptoms of Parkinson's disease include tremors (usually in the hands or fingers), rigidity (stiffness of the limbs and

Chapter 4: Basal Ganglia and Movement Quality

trunk), bradykinesia (slowness of movement), and postural instability (balance problems). These symptoms can make it difficult for individuals with Parkinson's disease to carry out daily activities and can significantly impact their quality of life.

In addition to motor symptoms, Parkinson's disease can also cause non-motor symptoms such as depression, anxiety, sleep disorders, and cognitive impairment.

Akinesia and Bradykinesia: Patients with Parkinson's disease show decreased activity and lack motivation and emotion. The patient shows a mask-like facial expression, a flexed trunk, neck, and arms, and a shuffling gait. Shuffling of the feet appears in addition to a lack of associated movement (arms do not swing while walking). Affected people have difficulty moving to a standing position from sitting. The slowness of action is also seen. *Pathology:* The loss of dopaminergic neurons in the substantia nigra compacta causes an increased (inhibitory) output from the basal ganglia. Increased inhibition of the thalamus can lead to less activation of the motor cortex and reduced voluntary movement.

Tremor: The resting tremor is another feature of Parkinson's disease. Patients' hand movements can be compared to using the thumb to roll a pill along the fingertips (pill-rolling tremor). The tremor is prominent when the hand is at rest. Typically, the resting tremor diminishes during voluntary movement.

Rigidity: The patient has increased muscle tone, "cogwheeling." Rigidity is about increased resistance to passive movement in all muscles. This muscle rigidity differs from muscle spasticity. This is because such rigidity is not associated with hyperreflexia, clonus, or clasp-knife responses.

Muscle Weakness: Muscle weakness is due to an increased inhibition output from the basal ganglia, leading to inhibition of the thalamus and, in turn, the somatomotor cortex. Decreased output from the somatomotor cortex leads to less activity in the pyramidal system, causing muscle weakness.

Visuoperceptual Deficits: The visuoperceptual deficit impedes action. For example, a therapist or carer intending to assist a person with ambulation often creates a visual block, and movement stops. People frequently report difficulties moving past visual movement blocks, like doorways. If a marker is placed on the floor, the person can use it as a cue for getting through the doorway. Why the marker does not serve as an additional visual block is not known. Late in the disease process, dementia may also develop.

Treatments:

Treatment for Parkinson's disease typically involves medications that increase dopamine levels in the brain, such as levodopa, as well as other medications that help manage symptoms. In some cases, surgery may be an option, such as deep brain stimulation (DBS), which involves implanting electrodes in the brain to help regulate abnormal brain activity. Physical therapy and exercise can also be helpful in managing motor symptoms and improving mobility and quality of life for individuals with Parkinson's disease.

Drug therapy: Drug therapy is used to interrupt basal ganglia circuits. L-DOPA supplements are used to stimulate both direct and indirect pathways of the basal ganglia (Fig. 4.6). D1 agonist can be used to stimulate the basal ganglia's direct pathway (Fig. 4.7).

Transplantation of fetal nigra graft: A surgical procedure is an alternative to drug therapy. Short-term benefits have been documented. However, further studies are needed to evaluate the long-term benefits. Studies have shown that fetal nigra grafts can be successfully transplanted into the striatum of humans and rodents. Transplantation of fetal nigra grafts can bring the level of dopamine to near normal twelve months after the graft. PET scans have shown that the cells are alive after the transplantation. They also showed that there was much less fluorodopa in the striatum before the transplantation. After an intracerebral ventricular injection of labeled L-DOPA, nerve terminals of dopaminergic fibers can take up fluorodopa.

L-DOPA corrects akinesia in Parkinson's disease

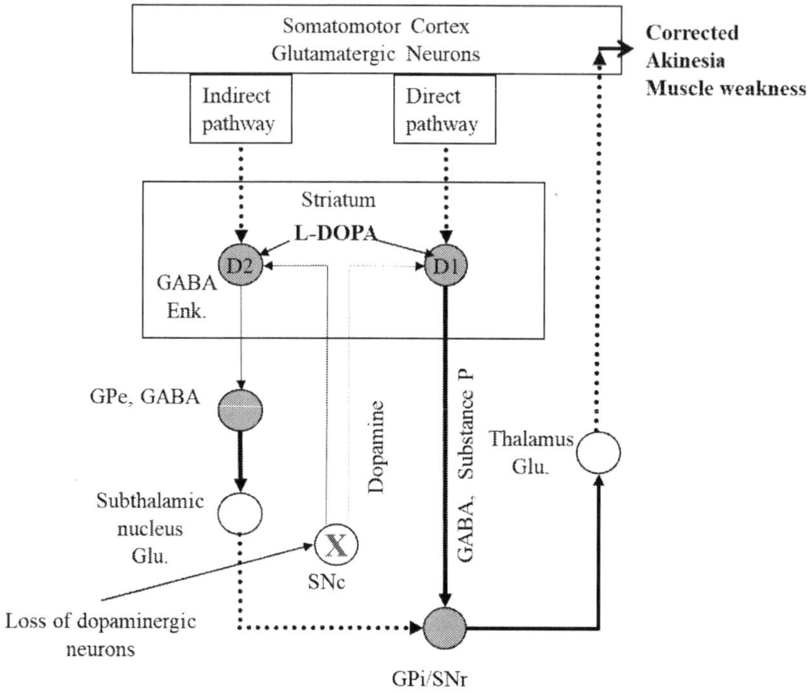

Figure 4.6. L-DOPA can alleviate Parkinson's symptoms. Administration of L-DOPA stimulates dopamine D1 and D2 receptors in the striatum. On the direct pathway, D1 receptor activation replaces the input of dopamine from the substantia nigra in the midbrain. Activation of the direct pathway inhibits the internal globus pallidus to the thalamus, as presented in Parkinson's disease. On the other hand, L-DOPA can inhibit the indirect basal ganglia pathway, leading to a decreased inhibitory effect from the internal globus pallidus to the thalamus.

Chapter 4: Basal Ganglia and Movement Quality

D1 agonist may correct Parkinson's symptoms

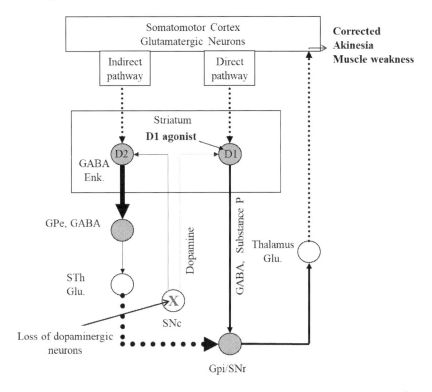

Figure 4.7. D1 agonist corrects Parkinson's symptoms. The figure shows a balance of inputs established in Parkinsonism following the administration of a selective D1 agonist. The D1 agonist can activate the direct basal ganglia pathway, leading to a decreased inhibitory effect from the internal globus pallidus to the thalamus, as presented in Parkinson's disease.

MPTP induced dopaminergic neuron lesion

MPTP (1-methyl-4-phenyl-1,2,3,6-tetrahydropyridine) is a neurotoxin that selectively destroys dopamine-producing neurons in the brain, including those in the substantia nigra. MPTP has been used extensively in animal models of Parkinson's disease to mimic the dopamine depletion that occurs in the disease.

MPTP is converted into a toxic metabolite called MPP+ (1-methyl-4-phenylpyridinium) by monoamine oxidase B (MAO-B) enzymes, which are highly expressed in dopamine-producing neurons. MPP+ accumulates in the neurons and causes oxidative stress and mitochondrial dysfunction, ultimately leading to cell death.

The destruction of dopamine-producing neurons by MPTP results in a depletion of dopamine in the brain, which leads to the motor symptoms of Parkinson's disease, including tremors, rigidity, bradykinesia, and postural instability (Fig. 4.8). These symptoms are similar to those observed in human Parkinson's disease and can be used to study the disease and test potential treatments.

Animal models of MPTP-induced dopaminergic neuron lesion and motor dysfunction have been used to investigate the pathophysiology of Parkinson's disease and to test potential therapies. Treatments that have been effective in these animal models include dopamine replacement therapy, such as levodopa, as well as neuroprotective agents that target oxidative stress and mitochondrial dysfunction.

Chapter 4: Basal Ganglia and Movement Quality

Overall, the MPTP-induced dopaminergic neuron lesion model has been a valuable tool for understanding the pathophysiology of Parkinson's disease and for developing and testing potential treatments.

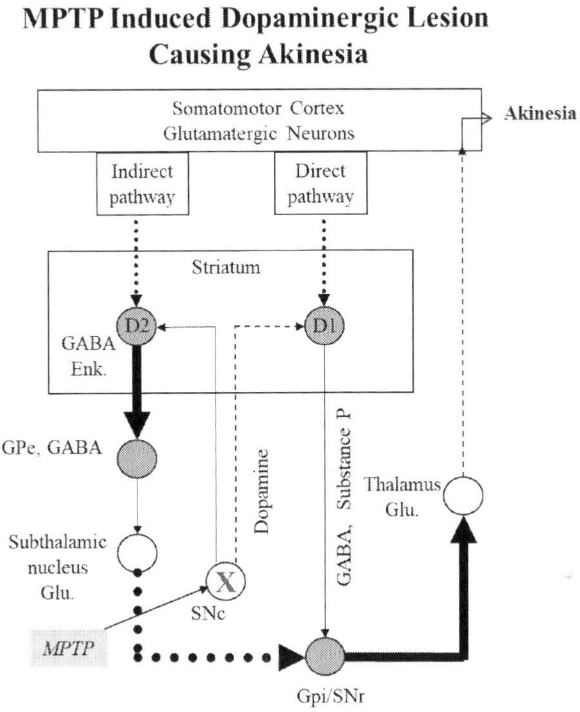

MPTP Induced Dopaminergic Lesion Causing Akinesia

Figure 4.8. Mechanism after an MPTP lesion to the dopaminergic neurons in the substantia nigra. The consequence is akinesia. MPTP is toxic to the dopaminergic neurons in the substantia nigra, which causes Parkinsonism. Degeneration of the dopaminergic projection from the substantia nigra pars compacta leads to underactivity in the direct pathway (thin arrow from the striatum to internal globus pallidus). It also leads to overactivity in the output of the indirect pathway from the subthalamic nucleus to the internal globus pallidus (thick open arrow). The result is excessive activity in the output neurons of the internal globus pallidus (thick-filled arrow) and reduced activity (akinesia) in the output neurons from the thalamus to the cortex.

Subthalamic Nucleus Lesion for treating advanced Parkinson's patients

Subthalamic nucleus (STN) lesion is a neurosurgical technique that has been used to treat Parkinson's disease (PD) since the 1990s. The procedure involves destroying a small area of the STN using heat, cold or electrical currents. The goal of the procedure is to reduce the abnormal electrical activity in the STN that contributes to the motor symptoms of PD (Fig. 4.9).

STN lesioning is typically reserved for patients with advanced PD who are no longer responding to medication or who are experiencing severe side effects from their medication. The procedure is not a cure for PD, but it can significantly improve motor symptoms such as tremors, rigidity, and bradykinesia. Patients who undergo STN lesioning may be able to reduce their medication dosage or even discontinue medication altogether.

The decision to pursue STN lesioning as a treatment option for PD is complex and requires careful consideration by both the patient and their healthcare team. The procedure carries some risks,

Chapter 4: Basal Ganglia and Movement Quality

including the potential for cognitive and speech impairment, and it is not appropriate for all patients with PD. Patients who are interested in STN lesioning should discuss the potential benefits and risks of the procedure with their doctor, and they should be evaluated by a multidisciplinary team of specialists with expertise in PD and neurosurgery.

Subthalamic nucleus lesion may correct Parkinson's symptoms

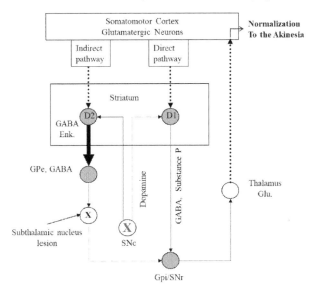

Figure 4.9. The above figure shows the mechanism of subthalamic nucleus lesions that can alleviate Parkinson's symptoms. In Parkinson's disease, the subthalamic nucleus is overactivated, which stimulates the inhibitory neurons in the globus pallidus; therefore, a consequence of akinesia. However, after the subthalamic nucleus lesion, the inhibition to the globus pallidus is reduced; therefore, a correction of akinesia.

Huntington's Disease

Huntington's disease is a progressive neuronal degenerative disease caused by a defective gene chromosome 4, which affects movement, mood, and cognitive skills. It mainly affects the striatum and cerebral cortex.

Symptoms

Huntington's disease (HD) is a rare, inherited neurodegenerative disorder that affects the brain. It is caused by a genetic mutation on chromosome 4 that leads to the production of an abnormal form of the huntingtin protein. This protein accumulates in the brain and causes damage to nerve cells, leading to the progressive deterioration of cognitive, motor, and psychiatric functions.

The symptoms of HD usually appear in adulthood, typically between the ages of 30 and 50. The earliest symptoms may include changes in mood, personality, and cognitive function, such as difficulty with memory, concentration, and decision-making. As the disease progresses, patients may experience involuntary movements, such as chorea (involuntary jerking or twitching), as well as difficulties with coordination, balance, and speech. Patients with HD may also develop psychiatric symptoms such as depression, anxiety, irritability, and impulsivity.

Chapter 4: Basal Ganglia and Movement Quality

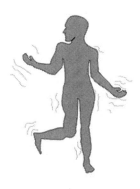

Figure 4.10. The hallmark symptom of Huntington's disease is uncontrolled movement of the arms, legs, head, face, and upper body. Huntington's chorea consists of involuntary, purposeless, irregular, jerky, and rapid movements.

The disease has striatum lesions affecting body movement and coordination. It is the progressive loss of medium spiny glutamatergic neurons in the striatum. These neurons are part of the indirect movement control pathway, which regulates fine movements. Genetically, the mutation is CAG (cytosine, adenine, guanine) trinucleotide repeated ten to thirty-five times.

The neural pathology of Huntington's disease is that a selective loss of the striatal GABA/enkephalinergic neurons occurs (Fig. 4.11). These neurons normally project to the external globus pallidus. Degeneration of these neurons results in increased inhibition of the subthalamic nucleus neurons. This decreases the signals from the basal ganglia and results in disinhibition of the motor thalamus.

The result is excessive output from the motor areas of the cerebral cortex.

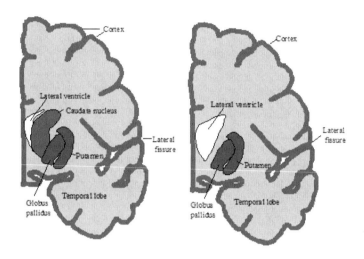

Figure 4.11. The transverse sections of two brains. Left, transverse section of normal brain with normal caudate; right, transverse section of a patient with Huntington's disease and severe caudate. On the left side, a normal brain with a normal caudate. The brain on the right side is from a patient with Huntington's disease showing severe caudate atrophy.

There is currently no cure for HD, and treatment is primarily focused on managing symptoms and improving quality of life. Medications may be used to manage psychiatric symptoms such as depression and anxiety, and physical therapy can help improve mobility and reduce the risk of falls. Genetic testing and counseling are also available for individuals with a family history of HD or who a

HD is a progressive and debilitating condition, and the course of the disease varies widely from person to person. Some individuals may experience a relatively slow progression of symptoms, while others may experience more rapid deterioration. However, with proper management and support, individuals with HD can maintain a good quality of life for many years.

Ballism

Ballism is a type of abnormal movement disorder that involves sudden, wild, and flinging movements of a limb or limbs. It is typically seen in the arms or legs, but can also occur in the trunk or neck. Ballism is a type of chorea, which is a neurological condition characterized by involuntary, irregular, and unpredictable movements.

The movements associated with ballism can be very forceful and can occur randomly or be triggered by certain movements. They can be repetitive or occur in bursts. The affected limb may swing in a wide arc, causing the individual to lose balance or fall.

Ballism is most commonly caused by damage to a part of the brain called the subthalamic nucleus, which is involved in the regulation of movement (Fig. 4.12). Conditions that can cause damage to this area of the brain include stroke, infection, and certain neurodegenerative disorders.

The treatment of ballism depends on the underlying cause. If it is caused by a reversible condition, such as medication-induced movement disorder, adjusting or discontinuing the medication may resolve the symptoms. In cases where the underlying cause cannot be reversed, medications that affect the levels of dopamine in the brain, such as antipsychotics or levodopa, may be used to manage the symptoms of ballism.

Overall, the management of ballism requires an individualized approach and should involve a healthcare team that includes a neurologist and physical therapist. With proper treatment and management, individuals with ballism can improve their quality of life and minimize the impact of the condition on their daily activities.

Chapter 4: Basal Ganglia and Movement Quality

Ballism: Subthalamic Lesion

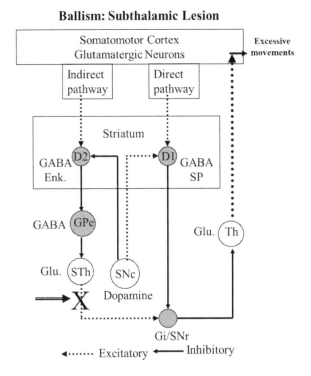

Figure 4.12. A subthalamic nucleus lesion causes ballism. The figure shows how a subthalamic nucleus lesion causes ballism. The lesion reduces the excitatory input from the subthalamic nucleus to the internal globus pallidus. As a result, less inhibition of the internal globus pallidus to the thalamus leads to more excitation of the somatomotor cortex. Thus, a person with ballism experiences extra and unwanted movements.

Stroke

A *stroke* is caused by a lack of blood supply to the brain and can be local or extensive, depending on which brain vessel is involved. It can be an *ischemic stroke, hemorrhagic stroke*, or *transient ischemic attack* (mini-stroke).

Stroke can cause motor dysfunction, which refers to a range of movement problems that can occur after a stroke. Motor dysfunction is a common symptom of stroke and can affect different parts of the body, depending on the location and severity of the stroke.

For example, if the stroke affects the motor cortex, it can cause weakness, paralysis, or difficulty with coordination and movement in one or more parts of the body, such as the arms, legs, or face. This can make it difficult to perform activities of daily living, such as dressing, eating, or walking.

If the stroke affects the basal ganglia, it can cause movement disorders such as tremors, rigidity, or difficulty with initiating and controlling movement, as seen in Parkinson's disease.

Rehabilitation is an important part of stroke treatment and may include physical therapy, occupational therapy, speech therapy, and other interventions aimed at improving motor function and quality of life.

Chapter 4: Basal Ganglia and Movement Quality

Internal Capsule Lesion

The internal capsule lies between the striatum and the thalamus inside the subcortical nuclei. It consists of numerous descending projections from the somatomotor cortex to the spinal cord. This is a crucial structure most of the descending nerve fibers from the motor cortex pass through. These include the corticospinal and corticobulbar tracts.

The vessel supplying the internal capsule is one common site of brain vascular accidents. Therefore, an internal capsule hemorrhage causes extensive muscle dysfunction.

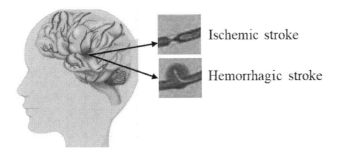

Figure 4.13. Stroke. The figure shows a hemorrhage caused by atherosclerosis in the internal capsule region of the brain, which can cause internal capsule lesions.

- *Motor dysfunction in the acute phase:* In severe cases, internal capsule hemorrhage can cause capsular hemiplegia and complete paralysis of the muscles involved. Symptoms of capsular hemorrhage are flaccid muscles on the contralateral side of the limbs. Muscle paralysis will be on the right side if the lesion on the internal capsule is on the left side. Typically, no reflexes are seen up to twelve hours after the stroke.

- *Motor dysfunction after acute phase:* A muscle hyper-reflexivity may be seen a week after an internal capsular lesion. Tendon jerks reappear, clonus may be seen, and muscle tone gradually increases. A clasp-knife reflex may be induced due to increased gamma motor neuron activity. Voluntary movement may recover progressively depending on the damage as well as the age of the patient.

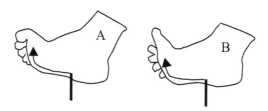

Figure 4.14. Babinski sign. The figure shows that the Babinski sign is negative (A) or the Babinski sign is positive (B).

Babinski's sign is a reflex response that is commonly used to assess the function of the nervous system, particularly the corticospinal tract. It is named after the French neurologist Joseph Babinski, who first described the sign in 1896.

Chapter 4: Basal Ganglia and Movement Quality

In a normal response, when the sole of the foot is stroked, the toes curl downward. This is known as a plantar reflex. However, in people with certain neurological conditions or damage to the corticospinal tract, the response may be abnormal. When the sole of the foot is stroked, the big toe moves upward, and the other toes fan out. This is known as a Babinski's sign or an up-going toe sign.

Babinski's sign is most commonly seen in people with damage to the upper motor neurons, such as in stroke, multiple sclerosis, spinal cord injury, or brain tumors. It can also be seen in newborns up to the age of 2 years, as their nervous system is still developing and the corticospinal tract is not fully myelinated.

Babinski's sign is an important clinical finding that can provide important information about the function of the nervous system. It is usually assessed as part of a neurological examination and can help to diagnose or rule out certain conditions. However, it should be interpreted in the context of other clinical findings and imaging studies, as it is not specific to any one condition.

Differences between Motor Cortex and Internal Capsule Lesions

Motor Cortex Lesions

A local motor defect is a feature of the cortical lesion, which is different from a major nerve fiber tract lesion, such as those occurring in internal capsule lesions. Because the cortical lesion is localized, the appearance of peripheral motor deficits is commonly localized. Furthermore, brain cortical lesions can cause high-level deficits, for example, dysphasia (language deficits).

Internal Capsule Lesions

As mentioned above, the internal capsule is formed by a collection of major fibers derived from the primary motor cortex, which project to the motor neurons in the brainstem and spinal cord. A lesion of the internal capsule causes many peripheral effects and, usually, no high-level deficits, such as dysphasia.

Chapter 4: Basal Ganglia and Movement Quality

The table shows the differences in motor dysfunction between cortex and internal capsule lesions

	Cortex Lesion Motor Dysfunction	**Internal Capsule Lesion Motor Dysfunction**
Location	In the outer layer (cortex) of the brain, just beneath the skull	In the deep part of the brain, between the cortex and the thalamus
Primary Motor Symptoms	Weakness or paralysis in specific parts of the body, depending on the location of the lesion in the cortex	Weakness or paralysis in specific parts of the body, depending on which part of the internal capsule is affected
Secondary Motor Symptoms	Difficulty with coordination and movement, including fine motor skills, gross motor skills, and gait	Difficulty with initiating and controlling movement, including spasticity, tremors, and rigidity
Babinski's Sign	May be present if the lesion is located in the precentral gyrus of the motor cortex	May be present if the lesion affects the corticospinal tract in the posterior limb of the internal capsule
Prognosis	Generally good, with recovery of function possible with rehabilitation and time	Recovery of function may be more difficult due to the location of the lesion and the potential for damage to the corticospinal tract
Treatment	Rehabilitation, such as physical therapy, occupational therapy, and speech therapy, to promote recovery of function	Rehabilitation, such as physical therapy, occupational therapy, and speech therapy, to promote recovery of function; surgery may be necessary in some cases

CHAPTER 5: SPINAL CORD REGULATES MOTOR FUNCTION

The spinal cord is a critical component of the nervous system that plays an important role in regulating motor function throughout the body. The spinal cord contains motor neurons, which are specialized cells that transmit signals from the brain to the muscles throughout the body. These signals, called motor commands, initiate muscle contractions that enable movement.

The spinal cord is divided into segments, with each segment corresponding to a specific area of the body. The cervical (neck) region of the spinal cord controls the upper body, including the arms, shoulders, and neck. The thoracic (chest) region of the spinal cord controls the trunk, while the lumbar (lower back) and sacral (pelvic) regions of the spinal cord control the legs, hips, and pelvic organs.

Motor function is regulated by a complex network of neurons within the spinal cord. This network, called the spinal reflex arc, is responsible for generating automatic responses to certain stimuli, such as the withdrawal reflex that occurs when a person touches a hot stove. This reflex arc allows for rapid responses to potentially dangerous situations without requiring input from the brain.

In addition to the reflex arc, the spinal cord also plays a crucial role in voluntary movement. When the brain sends a motor command down the spinal cord, it activates the appropriate motor neurons that connect to the relevant muscles. The motor neurons then transmit signals that cause the muscles to contract, resulting in movement.

Damage to the spinal cord can disrupt motor function by interfering with the transmission of signals between the brain and muscles. This can result in partial or complete paralysis, loss of sensation, and other motor control impairments. Rehabilitation after a spinal cord injury often involves physical therapy and other interventions to help individuals regain as much motor function and independence as possible.

SPINAL CORD

The spinal cord is an extension of the brain at the medulla oblongata area and ends in the lower back.

Anatomically, the spinal cord runs from the top of the first neck bone (the C1 vertebra) to the level of the first lumbar vertebra (L1). The spinal cord has two enlargements at the neck and lumbar regions.

The spinal cord lies inside the spinal column, surrounded by cerebrospinal fluid. The spinal column is made of vertebrae bones. Discs serve as shock absorbers for the spinal bones between the bodies of vertebral bones. These discs have an annulus fibrosus (tough outer layer) and nucleus pulposus.

The spinal cord has thirty-one pairs of spinal nerves. These spinal nerves exit the spinal cord via the intervertebral foramen. There are eight pairs of cervical nerves, twelve pairs of thoracic nerves, five pairs of lumbar nerves, and five pairs of sacral nerves. These are the peripheral nerves connecting the spinal cord to the upper and lower limbs and trunk.

The spinal cord receives sensory input responsible for motor control. Peripheral signals come into the spinal cord via peripheral nerves. The cell bodies providing sensation for the spinal nerve are located in the dorsal root ganglia. The dorsal horn of the spinal cord is responsible for receiving sensory information.

Any interruption of the spinal cord can result in a loss of motor function and sensation below that level.

Upper Motor Neurons

Upper motor neurons are a type of neuron that originate in the brain and are responsible for transmitting signals down to the spinal cord. These neurons play a crucial role in motor control and coordination of movements.

Chapter 5: Spinal Cord Regulates Motor Function

Upper motor neurons are located in the primary motor cortex, which is a region of the brain that is responsible for planning and executing movements. When the brain sends a motor command, it activates the appropriate upper motor neurons that project down to the spinal cord. These neurons synapse onto lower motor neurons, which then transmit signals to the muscles to initiate movement.

Damage to upper motor neurons can result in a variety of motor control impairments, including spasticity, muscle weakness, and difficulty with voluntary movements. For example, upper motor neuron lesions caused by stroke or other neurological conditions can result in hemiplegia or paralysis of one side of the body.

In addition to motor control, upper motor neurons also play a role in regulating reflexes and other involuntary movements. They help to modulate the activity of lower motor neurons and interneurons within the spinal cord to control muscle tone and maintain balance and posture.

Overall, upper motor neurons are an important component of the nervous system that are essential for the regulation and coordination of motor function throughout the body.

Lower Motor Neurons

Lower motor neurons are a type of neuron that are located within the spinal cord and are responsible for transmitting signals from the spinal cord to the muscles throughout the body. These neurons play a crucial role in motor control and the initiation of movements.

Lower motor neurons receive input from upper motor neurons and interneurons within the spinal cord. When activated, they transmit signals through their axons to the muscle fibers, causing them to contract and produce movement. The activation of lower motor neurons is what ultimately leads to the execution of voluntary movements and the control of muscle tone.

Damage to lower motor neurons can result in a variety of motor control impairments, including muscle weakness, atrophy, and hypotonia (reduced muscle tone). For example, lower motor neuron lesions caused by spinal cord injury or neurological conditions such as ALS (amyotrophic lateral sclerosis) can result in muscle weakness and paralysis.

Lower motor neurons are also responsible for regulating reflexes and other involuntary movements. They receive input from sensory neurons that detect changes in muscle length and tension, and they respond by causing the appropriate muscle contractions to maintain balance and posture.

Overall, lower motor neurons are an important component of the nervous system that are essential for the regulation and coordination of motor function throughout the body.

Distribution of the Lower Motor Neurons

Chapter 5: Spinal Cord Regulates Motor Function

The lower motor neurons are located in the anterior horn of the spinal cord and send the axons forming the spinal nerves.

Segments: The spinal cord can be divided into segments: cervical (C1–8), thoracic (T1–12), lumbar (L1–5), and sacral (S1–5).

Distribution: The distribution of lower motor neurons in the spinal cord varies. The cervical and lumbar enlargements contain many lower motor neurons because the cervical enlargement needs to supply the upper limbs, and the lumbar enlargement innervates the lower limbs. Cervical enlargement is at levels between C3 and T1 of the spinal cord. Lumbar enlargement is at levels between L1 and S3 of the spinal cord.

Topographic arrangements of lower motor neurons

The topographic arrangement of lower motor neurons refers to the organization of these neurons in the spinal cord, which is based on a somatotopic map. This map is a representation of the body on the spinal cord, where different regions of the body are represented in specific areas of the spinal cord.

The somatotopic map of the spinal cord can be divided into several regions, based on the location of the lower motor neurons that control movement of specific body parts. In general, the lower motor neurons that control movement of the upper limbs are located in the cervical region of the spinal cord, while the lower motor neurons that control movement of the lower limbs are located in the lumbar and sacral regions of the spinal cord.

Within each region, the lower motor neurons are organized in a specific way, based on the specific body part they control. For example, in the cervical region of the spinal cord, the lower motor neurons that control movement of the hand and fingers are located more laterally, while the lower motor neurons that control movement of the shoulder and upper arm are located more medially.

This topographic arrangement of lower motor neurons is important for the control and coordination of movements throughout the body. When an upper motor neuron sends a signal to a lower motor neuron, it activates a specific group of muscles that are controlled by that neuron. By organizing the lower motor neurons in a somatotopic map, the brain can efficiently control movement of different body parts, allowing for precise and coordinated movements. There is a topographic arrangement of lower motor neurons in the spinal cord where the neurons supplying the axial muscle lie in the medial part of the anterior horn of the spinal cord. The neurons supplying the distal muscles lie in the lateral part of the anterior horn of the spinal cord. Neurons supplying the flexor muscles lie in the dorsal part of the anterior horn of the spinal cord, and those innervating the extensor muscles lie in the ventral part of the anterior horn of the spinal cord.

Chapter 5: Spinal Cord Regulates Motor Function

Alpha Motor Neuron

Alpha motor neuron is a type of lower motor neurons that is responsible for transmitting signals from the spinal cord to the extrafusal muscle fibers, which are the muscle fibers responsible for generating force and movement.

Alpha motor neurons are located in the ventral horn of the gray matter in the spinal cord, and they are the primary efferent neurons that innervate skeletal muscles.

When an alpha motor neuron is activated, it causes the extrafusal muscle fibers that it innervates to *contract*, leading to movement of the associated body part. The activation of alpha motor neurons is under the control of upper motor neurons, which are located in the motor cortex of the brain and the brainstem. Upper motor neurons send signals down the spinal cord to activate the appropriate alpha motor neurons, leading to the *execution of voluntary movements*.

Alpha motor neurons are also responsible for regulating *muscle tone*, which is the amount of tension present in a muscle at rest. When alpha motor neurons are activated, they cause the extrafusal muscle fibers to contract and generate tension, which helps to maintain muscle tone and prevent atrophy.

Overall, alpha motor neurons play a crucial role in the control and coordination of voluntary movements and the maintenance of muscle tone. Damage to alpha motor neurons can result in a variety of motor control impairments, including muscle weakness, atrophy, and hypotonia. Rehabilitation after damage to alpha motor neurons often involves physical therapy and other interventions to help individuals regain as much motor function and independence as possible.

Alpha motor neuron injury

Injury to alpha motor neurons can have significant effects on motor function, as these neurons are responsible for transmitting signals from the spinal cord to the extrafusal muscle fibers, which are the muscle fibers responsible for generating force and movement.

Damage to alpha motor neurons can result from a variety of causes, including traumatic injuries such as spinal cord injury, degenerative diseases such as amyotrophic lateral sclerosis (ALS), and infectious or inflammatory conditions such as polio or autoimmune neuropathies.

The effects of alpha motor neuron injury depend on the severity and extent of the damage. In general, injury to alpha motor neurons can lead to muscle weakness, atrophy, and hypotonia (reduced muscle tone), which can result in difficulty with movement and impaired motor function.

Rehabilitation after alpha motor neuron injury often involves physical therapy and other interventions to help individuals regain as much motor function and independence as possible. This may include exercises to strengthen the remaining muscle fibers and

Chapter 5: Spinal Cord Regulates Motor Function

improve range of motion, as well as assistive devices such as braces or wheelchairs to help with mobility. In some cases, surgery may be necessary to repair or replace damaged neurons or to implant devices such as spinal cord stimulators to help control pain and improve motor function.

What inputs can influence alpha motor neuron?

Alpha motor neurons are the primary neurons responsible for controlling the contraction of skeletal muscle fibers. These neurons receive input from a variety of sources, including:

1. Upper motor neurons: These neurons originate in the brain and send axons down to the spinal cord, where they synapse onto alpha motor neurons. Upper motor neurons play a critical role in the control of voluntary movements and can influence the activity of alpha motor neurons.
2. Sensory neurons: Sensory neurons in the muscle, joints, and skin provide information to the central nervous system about the position and movement of the body. This information can influence the activity of alpha motor neurons, helping to regulate muscle contraction and maintain posture.
3. Interneurons: Interneurons are neurons that connect sensory neurons to motor neurons and can influence the activity of alpha motor neurons. They can also modulate the activity of other interneurons, helping to fine-tune the control of muscle contraction.

4. Reflexes: Reflexes are automatic responses to sensory input that can influence the activity of alpha motor neurons. For example, the stretch reflex is a reflex that occurs when a muscle is stretched, causing the muscle to contract in response.

Overall, the activity of alpha motor neurons is influenced by a complex interplay of inputs from sensory neurons, interneurons, and upper motor neurons, which helps to regulate the precise control of movement and maintain posture and balance.

Motor unit

A motor unit is a functional unit of the neuromuscular system that consists of a motor neuron and all the muscle fibers it innervates. When a motor neuron is activated by a signal from the nervous system, it causes all the muscle fibers in the motor unit to contract simultaneously. The number of muscle fibers in a motor unit can vary depending on the muscle and the degree of control required.

Motor units are classified based on several factors, including their size, contraction speed, and fatigue resistance. There are generally two types of motor units: slow-twitch (type I) motor units and fast-twitch (type II) motor units.

Slow-twitch motor units are smaller in size and contract more slowly, but they have a high resistance to fatigue and are used for sustained or endurance activities such as maintaining posture or running long distances.

Chapter 5: Spinal Cord Regulates Motor Function

Fast-twitch motor units, on the other hand, are larger in size and contract more quickly, but they fatigue more quickly as well. They are used for activities that require high force production in a short amount of time, such as lifting weights or sprinting.

The recruitment of motor units is controlled by the nervous system, which activates the motor units in a specific order depending on the force and speed required for the task at hand. As the force requirement increases, more motor units are recruited in a process called motor unit recruitment. The size principle of motor unit recruitment states that smaller motor units are recruited first, followed by larger motor units as the force requirement increases. This allows for fine control of muscle activity and efficient use of muscle fibers.

The table shows the characteristics of fast and slow motor units

Characteristic	Fast Motor Units	Slow Motor Units
Contraction speed	Fast	Slow
Fatigue resistance	Low	High
Recruitment threshold	High	Low
Motor neuron size	Large	Small
Force production	High	Low
Mitochondrial density	Low	High
Capillary density	Low	High
Myoglobin content	Low	High
Glycolytic capacity	High	Low
Oxidative capacity	Low	High

Motor Neuron Pool

A motor neuron pool refers to a group of motor neurons that are located in the spinal cord or brainstem and work together to control the contraction of a specific muscle or group of muscles.

Power and sustained muscle contraction: The central nervous system plays a vital role in generating the accumulated muscle fiber contraction. The central nervous system can recruit additional synergistic motor units if we need to increase power and sustained muscle contraction. The more muscle fibers accumulate in that motor unit, the higher the muscle contraction tension will become.

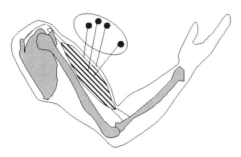

Figure 5.1. The figure shows a motor neuron pool defined as a group of alpha motor neurons innervating a single muscle.

The ratio of alpha motor neuron to muscle fiber

The nerve to muscle fiber ratio is an important factor that influences the accuracy and precision of movement. This ratio refers to the number of muscle fibers innervated by a single motor neuron. A lower ratio indicates that fewer muscle fibers are controlled by each motor neuron, leading to greater precision and accuracy of movement.

For example, muscles that require fine movements, such as those in the fingers and eyes, have a low nerve to muscle fiber ratio. This means that a smaller number of muscle fibers are controlled by each motor neuron, allowing for more precise and accurate control of movement.

In contrast, muscles that require more force and less precision, such as those in the legs, have a higher nerve to muscle fiber ratio. This means that a larger number of muscle fibers are controlled by each motor neuron, leading to less precision and accuracy of movement but more force production.

Therefore, the nerve to muscle fiber ratio is an important factor in determining the accuracy and precision of movement, and it varies depending on the type of muscle and the movement required.

Chapter 5: Spinal Cord Regulates Motor Function

The table shows differences between motor neuron pool and motor unit

	Motor neuron pool	Motor unit
Definition	All the motor neurons that innervate a particular muscle	A single alpha motor neuron and all the muscle fibers it innervates
Components	Alpha motor neurons and gamma motor neurons	A single alpha motor neuron and all the muscle fibers it innervates
Function	Regulate muscle contraction by controlling the number and firing patterns of alpha motor neurons	Regulate muscle contraction by synchronizing the firing of all the muscle fibers in the unit
Size	Varies depending on the muscle and degree of control required	Varies depending on the muscle and degree of control required
Number of components per unit	One motor neuron pool per muscle	Multiple motor units per muscle, each with its own alpha motor neuron and muscle fibers
Recruitment	Motor neurons in the pool are recruited in a specific order; depending on the force and speed required for the task at hand	Motor units are recruited in a specific order depending on the force and speed required for the task at hand, with smaller motor units recruited first followed by larger motor units

Gamma Motor Neuron

Gamma motor neurons are a type of motor neuron that innervates intrafusal muscle fibers within muscle spindles. Muscle spindles are sensory organs that are embedded in muscle fibers and are responsible for providing proprioceptive information about muscle length and tension to the central nervous system.

Gamma motor neurons innervate the intrafusal muscle. As a result, it increases the muscle spindles' tension and facilitates stretch reflexes. Furthermore, it adjusts the tension level of the intrafusal muscle fibers of the muscle spindle.

A gamma motor neuron has the opposite effect of an alpha motor neuron on Ia. (Alpha activation decreases Ia activity while gamma activation increases Ia activity.) It establishes the baseline activity in alpha motor neurons and helps regulate muscle length and tone.

In summary, gamma motor neurons are important for maintaining the sensitivity and accuracy of proprioceptive information by regulating the tension in intrafusal muscle fibers within muscle spindles.

Chapter 5: Spinal Cord Regulates Motor Function

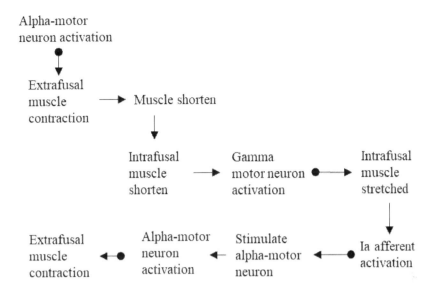

Figure 5.2. The flowchart above explains the operation of the gamma motor neurons between the spinal cord and the muscle, regulating muscle tension.

Gamma motor neuron syndrome, also known as gamma motor neuropathy, is a rare neurological disorder that affects the gamma motor neurons in the spinal cord. In gamma motor neuron syndrome, there is damage or dysfunction of the gamma motor neurons, which can lead to abnormalities in muscle tone and reflexes. The main symptoms of the condition include muscle weakness, stiffness, and spasticity, which can affect various parts of the body. The condition may also cause abnormalities in gait and posture, as well as other neurological symptoms such as sensory changes, tremors, or difficulty with coordination and balance.

Spinal Interneurons

Spinal excitatory and inhibitory interneurons play a crucial role in regulating motor function in the spinal cord. These interneurons act as intermediaries between sensory neurons that receive information from the body and motor neurons that control muscle movement.

Excitatory interneurons facilitate the transmission of signals from sensory neurons to motor neurons, resulting in muscle contraction. They are responsible for activating motor neurons that generate movement, such as the flexion of a limb.

On the other hand, inhibitory interneurons inhibit the activity of motor neurons and play an important role in regulating muscle activity. They can prevent muscle spasms or other unwanted movements by inhibiting the activity of motor neurons. For example, they may inhibit the activity of motor neurons responsible for maintaining muscle tone when a muscle is not in use.

Inhibitory interneurons also work together with excitatory interneurons to regulate the amplitude and timing of muscle contractions. This is important for precise movement control, such as when writing or playing a musical instrument.

Chapter 5: Spinal Cord Regulates Motor Function

Here are some examples:

1. When you walk, excitatory interneurons in the spinal cord activate motor neurons that control the muscles responsible for leg movement. Inhibitory interneurons simultaneously inhibit the activity of other motor neurons, preventing unwanted muscle contractions that could interfere with the coordinated movement of the legs.
2. When you touch a hot surface, sensory neurons in the skin send signals to the spinal cord. Excitatory interneurons then activate motor neurons that control the muscles responsible for quickly removing your hand from the hot surface. Inhibitory interneurons also play a role in this reflex response, inhibiting the activity of other motor neurons that could interfere with the desired movement.
3. During a sneeze, sensory neurons in the nose send signals to the spinal cord, which then activates excitatory interneurons that stimulate the muscles responsible for the sneeze reflex. Inhibitory interneurons also play a role, preventing the activation of other motor neurons that could cause unwanted movements during the reflex.
4. In individuals with spasticity, there is an imbalance between excitatory and inhibitory interneurons in the spinal cord, resulting in increased muscle tone and difficulty with movement. Treatments for spasticity often aim to restore this balance through medications or other interventions that target the spinal interneurons.

Overall, spinal excitatory and inhibitory interneurons work together to regulate motor function and maintain proper muscle control. Disruptions in this balance can lead to motor disorders or impairments.

Sensory Inputs related to motor control

Sensory inputs play an important role in motor control, providing information to the central nervous system about the position and movement of the body. There are several types of sensory inputs that are related to motor control:

1. Proprioceptive input: Proprioceptors are specialized sensory receptors located in muscles, tendons, and joints. They provide information about the position of body parts and the degree of muscle stretch, which is important for maintaining posture and controlling movement. For example, proprioceptive input allows us to walk without looking at our feet or to hold a cup without spilling the contents.
2. Cutaneous input: Cutaneous receptors are sensory receptors located in the skin that respond to touch, pressure, and temperature. They provide information about the surface of the skin and the objects in contact with it. This information is important for adjusting grip force, avoiding injury, and controlling movement in response to tactile stimuli.
3. Visual input: Visual input provides information about the environment and the position of the body relative to other

Chapter 5: Spinal Cord Regulates Motor Function

objects. It is important for guiding movements such as reaching, grasping, and walking.

4. Vestibular input: The vestibular system, located in the inner ear, provides information about head position and movement. This information is important for maintaining balance and posture.

All of these sensory inputs are integrated in the central nervous system to produce motor commands that control muscle activity. For example, the brain may use proprioceptive input to adjust muscle tone and maintain posture, cutaneous input to adjust grip force during grasping, visual input to guide reaching movements, and vestibular input to adjust balance during walking.

Sensory impairments can cause motor dysfunction because they disrupt the flow of information between the sensory and motor systems. Here are some examples:

1. Peripheral neuropathy: Peripheral neuropathy is a condition in which the nerves that transmit sensory information from the body to the central nervous system are damaged. This can result in sensory loss, such as numbness or tingling in the hands and feet. Without proper sensory input, individuals with peripheral neuropathy may experience difficulty with balance and coordination, as well as difficulty controlling fine motor movements such as writing or buttoning clothing.

2. Visual impairment: Visual impairment can impact motor function in a variety of ways. For example, individuals with reduced visual acuity may have difficulty judging distance or

accurately reaching for objects. They may also be more likely to trip or stumble, particularly in unfamiliar environments.

3. Vestibular dysfunction: The vestibular system plays a critical role in maintaining balance and posture. When the vestibular system is damaged, individuals may experience dizziness, vertigo, or difficulty with balance. This can make it difficult to walk, stand, or perform other movements that require balance and coordination.

4. Cerebellar ataxia: The cerebellum is an area of the brain that receives sensory input from the body and helps to coordinate movement. When the cerebellum is damaged, as in the case of cerebellar ataxia, individuals may experience difficulty with balance, coordination, and fine motor movements. For example, they may have trouble walking in a straight line or performing rapid alternating movements.

Overall, sensory impairments can have a significant impact on motor function, particularly when they involve the sensory systems that are critical for balance, coordination, and fine motor control.

Sensory nerve regulates motor function

Type Ia afferent fibers: These large-diameter sensory nerve fibers are found in muscle spindle fibers and are responsible for conveying information about muscle length and velocity to the central nervous system. They are highly sensitive to changes in muscle stretch and are critical for regulating precise movements.

Chapter 5: Spinal Cord Regulates Motor Function

Type Ib afferent fibers: These sensory nerve fibers are located within Golgi tendon organs and are sensitive to changes in tension within the tendon. They provide information about the force being generated by the muscle and help to prevent injury by regulating muscle activity during movement.

Type II afferent fibers: These sensory nerve fibers are also found in muscle spindle fibers and respond to changes in muscle length, but they are less sensitive than Type Ia fibers. They provide information about the position and movement of the body and help to regulate muscle tone.

Type III afferent fibers: These small-diameter sensory nerve fibers respond to changes in tension in muscle fibers and are found in muscle spindle fibers and Golgi tendon organs. They provide information about the force being generated by the muscles and help to regulate muscle activity during movement.

Type IV afferent fibers: These small-diameter sensory nerve fibers transmit pain and temperature information from the body to the central nervous system. They can be activated by a variety of stimuli and contribute to the experience of pain.

Overall, these different types of sensory nerve fibers work together to provide the central nervous system with a continuous stream of information about the position, movement, and force generated by the body during motor activities. This information is critical for regulating movements in response to changes in the environment or the body and for preventing injury during movement.

Table shows the neural afferent involved in motor control

Property	Group 1 Nerve Fiber Ia	Group 1 Nerve Fiber Ib	Group II Nerve Fiber
Fiber Diameter	Large (12-20 microns)	Large (12-20 microns)	Medium (6-12 microns)
Conduction Velocity	Fast (70-120 m/s)	Fast (30-70 m/s)	Medium (20-40 m/s)
Origin	Muscle spindle (primary afferent)	Golgi tendon organ (secondary afferent)	Secondary afferent
Function	Conveys information about muscle length and rate of change of length (velocity)	Conveys information about muscle tension (force)	Conveys information about muscle length and tension
Synapse Location	Alpha motor neuron dendrites (monosynaptic)	Interneurons (polysynaptic)	Interneurons (polysynaptic)
Role in Motor Control	Regulates muscle contraction by adjusting the sensitivity of the muscle spindle via gamma motor neurons.	Contributes to the autogenic inhibition reflex, which reduces muscle tension and prevents damage to the muscle.	Contributes to muscle length and tension regulation via feedback to the central nervous system.

Chapter 5: Spinal Cord Regulates Motor Function

Superficial sensation influences motor control

Superficial sensation plays an important role in movement control by providing information about the external environment and the position of the body in space. Superficial sensation refers to the sense of touch, pressure, temperature, and pain that is transmitted from the skin and other superficial tissues to the central nervous system. This information is integrated with other sensory inputs, such as proprioception and vision, to guide movement and maintain balance.

The sensory receptors responsible for detecting superficial sensation are located in the skin and include various types of mechanoreceptors, thermoreceptors, and nociceptors. Mechanoreceptors respond to mechanical stimulation, such as pressure and vibration, while thermoreceptors respond to changes in temperature, and nociceptors respond to noxious stimuli, such as injury or inflammation.

During movement, information from superficial sensation is used to guide the movement of the limbs and body in space. For example, when reaching for an object, the sense of touch and pressure from the fingers is used to guide the movement and adjust the grip on the object. Similarly, when walking on a rough or uneven surface, information from the soles of the feet is used to adjust the gait and maintain balance.

Disruptions to superficial sensation can lead to difficulties with movement control and balance. For example, individuals with peripheral neuropathy, which is a condition that affects the peripheral nerves responsible for transmitting sensation, may experience difficulties with balance and coordination due to the loss of sensation in their feet and hands.

Therefore, superficial sensation is an important component of movement control and plays a critical role in guiding movement and maintaining balance during daily activities.

Spinothalamic pathway

The spinothalamic pathway is a neural pathway that plays an important role in transmitting superficial sensation, such as pain and temperature, from the skin and other superficial tissues to the brain.

The spinothalamic pathway begins with the activation of nociceptors and thermoreceptors in the skin and other superficial tissues. These sensory receptors send signals through small-diameter Type III and Type IV sensory nerve fibers to the dorsal horn of the spinal cord, where they synapse with second-order neurons. The second-order neurons then cross over to the opposite side of the spinal cord and ascend through the spinothalamic tract to the thalamus.

Once in the thalamus, the spinothalamic pathway synapses with third-order neurons that project to the somatosensory cortex, where the sensations are perceived and localized. The spinothalamic pathway is also involved in reflexive responses to noxious stimuli, such as the withdrawal reflex.

Disruptions to the spinothalamic pathway can lead to alterations in superficial sensation, including pain, temperature, and tactile perception. For example, damage to the spinothalamic pathway can result in conditions such as central pain syndrome or peripheral neuropathy, which can lead to chronic pain or loss of sensation.

In summary, the spinothalamic pathway is an important neural pathway involved in the transmission of superficial sensation, including pain and temperature, from the skin and other superficial tissues to the brain. This pathway is critical for the perception and localization of superficial sensation, as well as for reflexive responses to noxious stimuli.

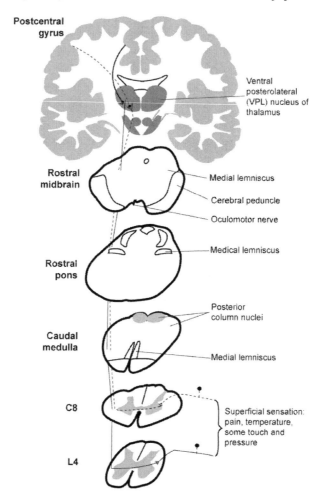

Figure 5.3. Spinothalamic pathway for superficial sensation inputs. The figure shows the spinothalamic pathway. The superficial sensation goes to the somatosensory cortex via the spinothalamic pathway: pain, temperature, pressure, and general touch.

Chapter 5: Spinal Cord Regulates Motor Function

Impairment of superficial sensation can lead to motor dysfunction in several ways:

1. Loss of tactile sensation: Tactile sensation is important for guiding movement and adjusting grip force. When there is a loss of tactile sensation due to damage to peripheral nerves, individuals may have difficulty controlling their movements and may be more prone to dropping objects or losing their balance.

2. Loss of proprioception: Proprioception is the sense of the position and movement of our body parts. Superficial sensation provides important feedback to the proprioceptive system, allowing us to adjust our movements based on the position of our limbs and joints. When there is a loss of superficial sensation, such as in peripheral neuropathy, individuals may have difficulty with movement control and may be more prone to falls.

3. Impaired pain sensation: Pain is an important warning signal that helps us avoid injury. When there is an impairment in superficial pain sensation, such as in diabetic neuropathy, individuals may continue to engage in activities that cause tissue damage, leading to further motor dysfunction.

4. Impaired temperature sensation: Temperature sensation is important for regulating body temperature and responding to changes in the environment. When there is an impairment in superficial temperature sensation, such as in peripheral neuropathy, individuals may be less able to regulate their body

temperature and may have difficulty responding to changes in the environment, leading to motor dysfunction.

Therefore, impairment of superficial sensation can lead to motor dysfunction by disrupting the ability to perceive and respond to sensory information from the environment, as well as by disrupting the feedback loop between sensory information and motor output.

Deep sensation involved in the regulation of motor function

Deep sensation plays an important role in the regulation of motor function. Deep sensation is the perception of stimuli arising from within the body, such as joint position, muscle length, and muscle tension. This information is carried by sensory neurons having proprioceptors and is essential for the maintenance of balance, coordination, and posture.

There are several types of proprioceptors that provide information about different aspects of movement and position:

1. Muscle spindles: These are specialized muscle fibers that detect changes in muscle length and velocity. They provide information about the position of the limbs and the speed and direction of movement.
2. Golgi tendon organs: These are sensory receptors located in tendons that detect changes in muscle tension. They provide information about the force being applied to a muscle and help to regulate muscle contraction.

Chapter 5: Spinal Cord Regulates Motor Function

3. Joint receptors: These are sensory receptors located in the joint capsules that provide information about joint position and movement. They play an important role in maintaining joint stability and coordinating movement.

The information provided by deep sensation is integrated with other sensory inputs, such as visual and vestibular input, to maintain balance and coordination during movement. For example, during walking, proprioceptive input from the feet and legs is integrated with visual input to adjust stride length and maintain balance.

Impairment of deep sensation can lead to motor dysfunction in several ways. For example, damage to muscle spindles can lead to difficulty in adjusting movement and grip force, while damage to joint receptors can lead to joint instability and difficulty in coordinating movement. Impairment of deep sensation can also affect postural control, leading to difficulty in maintaining balance and increased risk of falls.

Therefore, deep sensation plays a critical role in the regulation of motor function and maintaining balance, coordination, and posture.

Medial lemniscus pathway

The medial lemniscus pathway is one of the major pathways involved in the transmission of deep sensation information to the brain.

The medial lemniscus pathway begins in the periphery with the sensory receptors (muscle spindles, Golgi tendon organs, joint receptors) and their associated sensory neurons. The axons of these sensory neurons then travel through the dorsal root ganglia and into the spinal cord. Once in the spinal cord, the sensory axons synapse with second-order neurons in the dorsal column nuclei.

The axons of the second-order neurons then cross over to the opposite side of the brainstem in a region called the medial lemniscus. The axons continue to ascend through the brainstem and into the thalamus, where they synapse with third-order neurons. Finally, the axons of the third-order neurons project to the primary somatosensory cortex in the parietal lobe, where they are processed and integrated with other sensory information.

The medial lemniscus pathway is responsible for the transmission of *proprioceptive* and *tactile* information, which is essential for motor function. The pathway provides information about limb and joint position, muscle length, and muscle tension, which are critical for coordinating movement and maintaining balance and posture.

Damage to the medial lemniscus pathway can result in impaired deep sensation, leading to motor dysfunction. For example, damage to the pathway can lead to difficulties with limb and joint position sense, muscle coordination, and balance control.

In summary, the medial lemniscus pathway plays a critical role in the transmission of deep sensation information to the brain, which is essential for the regulation of motor function. The pathway provides information about limb and joint position, muscle length, and muscle tension, which are critical for coordinating movement and maintaining balance and posture.

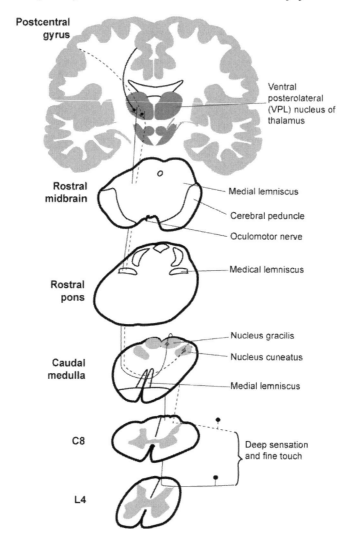

Figure 5.4. The medial lemniscus pathway for the inputs of deep sensation and fine touch.

Chapter 5: Spinal Cord Regulates Motor Function

Spinocerebellar pathway involved in motor control

The spinocerebellar pathway is another major pathway involved in the transmission of deep sensation information to the brain, specifically to the cerebellum.

The spinocerebellar pathway begins with the sensory receptors (muscle spindles, Golgi tendon organs, and joint receptors) and their associated sensory neurons in the periphery. The axons of these sensory neurons enter the spinal cord and synapse with second-order neurons in the dorsal horn of the spinal cord.

The axons of the second-order neurons then cross over to the opposite side of the spinal cord and ascend to the cerebellum via the spinocerebellar tract. There are two main pathways within the spinocerebellar tract: the dorsal spinocerebellar tract and the ventral spinocerebellar tract.

The dorsal spinocerebellar tract conveys information about the position and movement of the lower limbs and trunk. The ventral spinocerebellar tract conveys information about the position and movement of the upper limbs.

The spinocerebellar pathway provides the cerebellum with information about the position and movement of the limbs, which is critical for the coordination of movement and the maintenance of balance and posture. The cerebellum uses this information to adjust muscle activity and refine movement patterns.

Impairment of the spinocerebellar pathway can result in motor dysfunction, including difficulty with coordination, balance, and posture. For example, damage to the pathway can lead to ataxia, which is characterized by uncoordinated movements and a lack of balance control.

Therefore, the spinocerebellar pathway is another important pathway involved in the transmission of deep sensation information to the brain, specifically to the cerebellum. The pathway provides the cerebellum with information about the position and movement of the limbs, which is critical for the coordination of movement and the maintenance of balance and posture. Impairment of the pathway can result in motor dysfunction, including difficulty with coordination, balance, and posture.

Muscle twitching

Muscle twitching, also known as fasciculation, is characterized by the involuntary contraction or twitching of muscle fibers. It can occur in any muscle in the body, but is most commonly felt in the arms, legs, or face.

Muscle twitches are often described as a subtle, rapid movement that is not forceful enough to cause movement of the limb or body part. They may feel like a slight tingling or a tickling sensation under the skin. In some cases, muscle twitches can be seen on the

Chapter 5: Spinal Cord Regulates Motor Function

surface of the skin as small, involuntary muscle contractions or flickers.

Muscle twitches can occur randomly or may be triggered by certain actions or conditions, such as stress, anxiety, caffeine, or dehydration. They may also occur as a symptom of an underlying medical condition, such as nerve damage, electrolyte imbalances, or neurological disorders.

While muscle twitches can be uncomfortable or annoying, they are usually not a cause for concern and will resolve on their own. However, if muscle twitching is accompanied by other symptoms, such as weakness, numbness, or pain, it is important to seek medical attention to determine the underlying cause.

MUSCLES

Muscle spindle

A muscle spindle is a sensory organ found within skeletal muscles that is responsible for detecting changes in muscle length and tension. Muscle spindles play a critical role in proprioception, which is the sense of the body's position and movement in space.

Each muscle spindle is made up of specialized muscle fibers called intrafusal muscle fibers, which are surrounded by sensory nerve endings called proprioceptors. When the muscle spindle is stretched, the proprioceptors are activated, sending signals to the central nervous system that provide information about the position and movement of the body.

Muscle spindles are particularly important for maintaining posture, balance, and coordination during movement. They help to regulate muscle tone, which is the degree of tension in a muscle at rest, and they provide feedback to the central nervous system about changes in muscle length and tension, allowing for adjustments to be made to movement patterns.

The sensitivity of muscle spindles is regulated by gamma motor neurons, which are specialized motor neurons that innervate the intrafusal muscle fibers. When the muscle contracts, gamma motor neurons cause the intrafusal muscle fibers to contract as well, helping to maintain sensitivity to changes in muscle length.

Overall, muscle spindles are essential for the control of movement and the maintenance of posture and balance, providing the central nervous system with critical information about the position and movement of the body in space.

Intrafusal muscle fibers

Intrafusal muscle fibers are specialized muscle fibers located within muscle spindles, which are sensory organs found in skeletal muscles. Muscle spindles are responsible for detecting changes in muscle length and sending this information to the central nervous system to help regulate muscle contraction.

Intrafusal muscle fibers are surrounded by sensory nerve endings called proprioceptors, which detect changes in muscle length and tension. These proprioceptors, in turn, send signals to the central nervous system, providing information about the position and movement of the body.

There are two main types of intrafusal muscle fibers: nuclear bag fibers and nuclear chain fibers. Nuclear bag fibers have large, rounded central regions called bags, while nuclear chain fibers have elongated, chain-like central regions.

In order for muscle spindles to function properly, both types of intrafusal muscle fibers must be able to contract and stretch in response to changes in muscle length. This is accomplished through specialized sensory and motor neurons called gamma motor neurons, which innervate the intrafusal muscle fibers.

Overall, intrafusal muscle fibers play an important role in proprioception and the regulation of muscle tone, helping to maintain posture and perform movements with accuracy and precision.

Extrafusal muscle fibers

Extrafusal muscle fibers are the main skeletal muscle fibers responsible for generating force and movement in the body. They are so named because they are located outside of the muscle spindle, which is a sensory organ that detects changes in muscle length and sends information to the central nervous system.

Extrafusal muscle fibers are innervated by alpha motor neurons, which are located in the spinal cord and are part of the lower motor neuron system. When an alpha motor neuron is activated, it sends an electrical signal down its axon to the extrafusal muscle fibers it innervates, causing them to contract.

The contraction of extrafusal muscle fibers is responsible for generating the force required to move the skeleton and perform tasks such as lifting, walking, and running. The strength and speed of muscle contraction depend on a variety of factors, including the number and firing rate of activated motor units, the type of muscle fibers involved, and the level of neural input to the motor neurons.

Overall, extrafusal muscle fibers play a crucial role in the voluntary control of movement and are essential for maintaining posture, performing skilled movements, and engaging in physical activity.

Sustained voluntary muscle contraction

Sustained voluntary muscle contraction, also known as tonic contraction, involves the activation of muscle fibers for a prolonged period of time, without relaxation. This type of contraction is used for tasks such as maintaining posture, holding objects, and supporting body weight. The mechanism of sustained voluntary muscle contraction involves several processes, including:

1. Recruitment of motor units: Motor units are the functional units of muscle contraction, consisting of a single motor neuron and the muscle fibers it innervates. During sustained contraction, additional motor units are recruited to maintain force output and counteract fatigue.
2. Activation of type II muscle fibers: Type II muscle fibers are fast-twitch fibers that are capable of generating high levels of force. During sustained contraction, type II muscle fibers are activated to help maintain force output.
3. Activation of the stretch reflex: The stretch reflex, also known as the myotatic reflex, is activated during sustained contraction to help maintain muscle tone and prevent excessive stretching of the muscle.

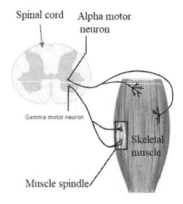

Figure 5.5. Sustained muscle contraction involved in alpha motor neurons, muscle spindle, and gamma motor neurons

Overall, sustained voluntary muscle contraction is a complex process that involves the recruitment of motor units, activation of type II muscle fibers, activation of the stretch reflex, maintenance of calcium levels, and energy production. The ability to sustain voluntary muscle contraction is essential for many daily activities, and it is dependent on the coordination of multiple physiological processes.

Golgi Tendon Organ

The Golgi tendon organ (GTO) is a sensory receptor located at the junction of skeletal muscle fibers and their tendons. It plays a crucial role in regulating motor function by providing sensory feedback to the central nervous system about the tension generated in a muscle during contraction.

Chapter 5: Spinal Cord Regulates Motor Function

The GTO senses changes in tension and stretch within a muscle, and sends information to the central nervous system via sensory neurons. This feedback mechanism allows the body to regulate muscle force and prevent overexertion or injury. For example, if a muscle is generating too much force, the GTO will signal the nervous system to decrease muscle contraction, thus preventing damage to the muscle or tendon.

When tension is applied to a muscle, the Ib fibers in the GTO are stimulated and send signals to the spinal cord. This initiates the Golgi tendon reflex, causing the muscle to relax and preventing it from over-contracting or overstretching.

The Ib fibers also play a role in proprioception, which is the sense of the body's position and movement in space. The information provided by Ib fibers helps the central nervous system to maintain accurate body position and movement control.

Therefore, the Golgi tendon organ is an important sensory receptor that helps to regulate motor function by providing feedback on muscle tension and stretch. Its role in the control of muscle force and posture highlights its importance in maintaining proper movement and preventing injury.

NEUROMUSCULAR CONTROL

The neuromuscular system is involved in movement control, including muscle activation patterns, motor unit recruitment, and proprioception.

The neuromuscular system plays a crucial role in movement control by integrating sensory information with motor commands to produce smooth and coordinated movements. Here are some key aspects of the neuromuscular system involved in movement control:

1. Muscle activation patterns: When a muscle contracts, it generates force by shortening its length. The pattern of muscle activation required for movement control depends on the task being performed. For example, to lift a heavy object, the muscles must generate a high level of force and be activated in a coordinated manner. In contrast, for more delicate movements such as typing on a keyboard, the muscles must generate low levels of force and be activated in a precise and controlled manner.

2. Motor unit recruitment: Muscles are made up of individual motor units, each of which consists of a motor neuron and the muscle fibers it innervates. Motor unit recruitment refers to the process by which motor neurons activate specific motor units to produce a desired level of muscle force. During movement

Chapter 5: Spinal Cord Regulates Motor Function

control, motor unit recruitment is regulated by the nervous system based on the level of force required for the task.

3. Proprioception: Proprioception refers to the sense of limb position and movement that is provided by receptors in the muscles, tendons, and joints. This information is used by the nervous system to regulate muscle activation and ensure accurate movement control. For example, when reaching for an object, the nervous system uses proprioceptive information to adjust the activation of the muscles in the arm and hand to produce a smooth and accurate movement.

4. Feedback mechanisms: The neuromuscular system also uses feedback mechanisms to monitor movement and make adjustments as needed. For example, when walking on an uneven surface, the nervous system uses sensory feedback from the feet and legs to adjust muscle activation and maintain balance. Similarly, during fine motor tasks such as handwriting, the nervous system uses sensory feedback from the fingers to adjust muscle activation and ensure accurate movement control.

Overall, the neuromuscular system plays a crucial role in movement control by integrating sensory information with motor commands to produce smooth and coordinated movements. Understanding the different aspects of the neuromuscular system involved in movement control can help guide the development of rehabilitation strategies for individuals with movement disorders.

Motor Reflex

Golgi tendon reflex

The Golgi tendon reflex is a reflexive response that occurs when the Golgi tendon organ (GTO), a sensory receptor located at the junction of skeletal muscle fibers and their tendons, is stimulated by excessive tension. The Golgi tendon reflex is a protective mechanism that helps to prevent muscle damage and maintain proper muscle tone.

The Golgi tendon reflex helps to prevent muscle damage by limiting the amount of tension that can be generated in a muscle. It is important for maintaining proper muscle tone and preventing overstretching or over-contraction of muscles. The Golgi tendon reflex is also thought to be involved in the control of posture and movement, as it provides sensory feedback to the central nervous system about the state of muscle tension.

The Golgi tendon reflex is one of several reflexes involved in the regulation of muscle tone and movement control. Other reflexes include the stretch reflex and the flexor withdrawal reflex. These reflexes all involve sensory input and spinal cord circuits, and help to ensure proper muscle function and movement control.

Chapter 5: Spinal Cord Regulates Motor Function

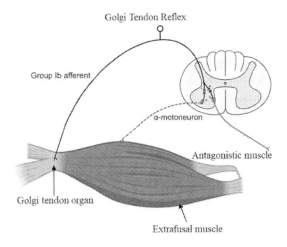

Figure 5.6. Golgi tendon reflex to prevent muscle injury by over-strengthening and maintain proper muscle tone.

Components of Golgi tendon reflex

The Golgi tendon reflex is a protective mechanism that uses signals from Ib sensory fibers to inhibit the activity of alpha motor neurons and prevent excessive contraction of extrafusal muscle fibers in response to excessive tension. This reflex prevents muscle from being damaged by excessive tension.

Ib sensory fibers are nerves that are connected to the Golgi tendon organ, which is a receptor that detects excessive tension in a muscle. When the GTO is stimulated by excessive tension, the Ib fibers send a signal to the spinal cord. In the spinal cord, the Ib fibers connect to inhibitory interneurons, which release a chemical that stops alpha motor neurons from activating the muscle.

Alpha motor neurons are nerves that cause the muscle to contract.

Extrafusal muscle fibers are the fibers in the muscle that actually contract and generate force.

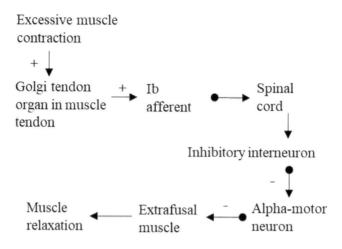

Figure 5.7. Flowchart for the process of the Golgi tendon reflex.

Stretch Reflex

The stretch reflex also known as the knee-jerk reflex or myotatic reflex, is a reflexive response of the muscle to an external stimulus that causes it to stretch. This reflex is a protective mechanism that helps to maintain muscle tone and prevent injury by quickly contracting a muscle when it is stretched too far

The stretch reflex is a very rapid response, with contraction occurring within a few milliseconds of the stretch stimulus. It is also

Chapter 5: Spinal Cord Regulates Motor Function

a monosynaptic reflex, meaning that it involves only one synapse between sensory and motor neurons.

The stretch reflex is important for maintaining posture and balance, as well as for performing rapid and coordinated movements. Also, an antigravity nerve feedback loop regulates the stretch reflex.

Here are the general steps of the muscle stretch reflex test:

1. The patient is seated or lying down comfortably, with the muscle to be tested relaxed.
2. The clinician applies a quick and brief stretch to the muscle by tapping it with a reflex hammer or by manually stretching it.
3. The stretch should be brief and not overly forceful, as this can elicit other reflexes and interfere with the results.
4. The examiner observes the muscle's response to the stretch, looking for a reflexive contraction of the muscle.
5. The examiner can then grade the reflex on a scale from 0 to 4, with 0 indicating no response and 4 indicating a very brisk response.

The clinician can perform the stretch reflex test on multiple muscles to assess the patient's overall reflexes.

The process of the stretch reflex involves several steps, including:

1. Stretch: The muscle spindle, a sensory receptor located within the muscle fibers, is stretched due to a sudden lengthening of the muscle.
2. Activation of sensory neurons: The stretching of the muscle spindle activates sensory neurons, specifically type Ia afferents, which travel through the dorsal root ganglia and into the spinal cord.
3. Excitation of alpha motor neurons: The sensory neurons synapse directly with alpha motor neurons in the spinal cord that innervate the same muscle.
4. Contraction of extrafusal muscle fibers: The excitation of the alpha motor neurons causes the extrafusal muscle fibers, which are responsible for generating force and movement, to contract.
5. Inhibition of antagonist muscles: The stretch reflex also activates inhibitory interneurons in the spinal cord, which inhibit the alpha motor neurons that control the antagonist muscles, preventing them from contracting and interfering with the reflexive contraction of the stretched muscle.

Chapter 5: Spinal Cord Regulates Motor Function

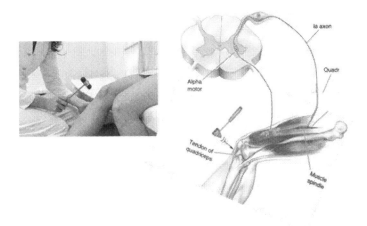

Figure 5.8. Test of a muscle stretch reflex.

Overall, the stretch reflex is a rapid and automatic response that helps to maintain muscle tone and prevent injury by quickly contracting a muscle in response to sudden stretching. The stretch reflex is an important component of the body's neuromuscular control system, and it is involved in maintaining posture, balance, and coordinated movement.

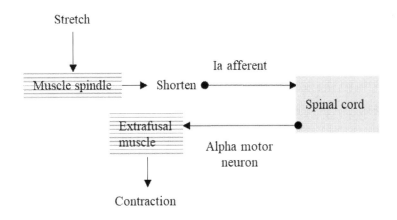

Figure 5.9. The stretch reflex process.

Clasp-Knife Reflex

The clasp-knife reflex is a type of reflexive response that occurs when a muscle is passively stretched, similar to the stretch reflex. However, the clasp-knife reflex is characterized by an initial resistance to the stretch, followed by a sudden release or "giving way" of the muscle.

The clasp-knife reflex is thought to be caused by the activation of stretch-sensitive neurons, called muscle spindles, located in the muscle being stretched. When a muscle is stretched, the muscle spindle is also stretched, and this activates sensory neurons that transmit signals to the spinal cord. In response, the spinal cord sends signals back to the muscle via alpha motor neurons, causing the muscle to contract and resist the stretch.

However, in the case of the clasp-knife reflex, the resistance to the stretch suddenly gives way or "gives" after a certain point, leading to a sudden decrease in resistance. This is thought to be caused by the activation of inhibitory interneurons in the spinal cord that are stimulated by the same stretch-sensitive neurons that activate the alpha motor neurons. The inhibitory interneurons cause the alpha motor neurons to stop firing, leading to the sudden relaxation of the muscle and the giving way that characterizes the clasp-knife reflex.

The clasp-knife reflex is commonly observed in patients with upper motor neuron lesions, such as those caused by stroke or spinal cord injury. It is thought to be a sign of increased muscle tone or spasticity, which can result from damage to the descending pathways that normally inhibit the activity of alpha motor neurons. The clasp-knife reflex is not the same as the Golgi tendon reflex, which is a protective mechanism that prevents excessive tension in a muscle.

While both the Golgi tendon reflex and the clasp-knife reflex involve sensory input and spinal cord circuits, they are different reflexes with different underlying mechanisms and effects on muscle tone. The Golgi tendon reflex is a protective reflex that helps to prevent muscle damage, while the clasp-knife reflex is a pathological reflex associated with spasticity.

Reciprocal Inhibition Reflex

Reciprocal inhibition reflex is a neurological reflex that occurs when a muscle is voluntarily contracted. It involves the inhibition of antagonist muscles that would otherwise oppose or interfere with the contraction of the agonist muscle.

During voluntary muscle contraction, both the agonist muscle (the muscle that is contracting) and the antagonist muscle (the muscle that opposes the contraction) receive signals from the nervous system. In reciprocal inhibition, the signal to the antagonist muscle is inhibited, allowing the agonist muscle to contract more effectively.

The reflex is mediated by the nervous system and involves the activation of inhibitory interneurons in the spinal cord. These interneurons are activated by sensory signals from muscle spindles and other sensory receptors, and they inhibit the motor neurons that innervate the antagonist muscle. This inhibition allows the agonist muscle to contract more effectively, without interference from the antagonist muscle.

Reciprocal inhibition reflex is an important mechanism for coordinating muscle activity and movement. It helps to ensure that movements are smooth and efficient, without unnecessary opposition or interference from antagonist muscles. The reflex is involved in many everyday activities, such as walking, running, and reaching, and it is essential for normal movement and function.

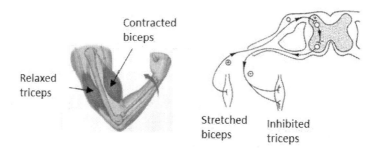

Figure 5.10. The figure shows an example of the reciprocal inhibition reflex. So it is that it stimulates one muscle contraction (biceps) and leads to the opposing muscle or antagonist muscle relaxation (triceps).

Chapter 5: Spinal Cord Regulates Motor Function

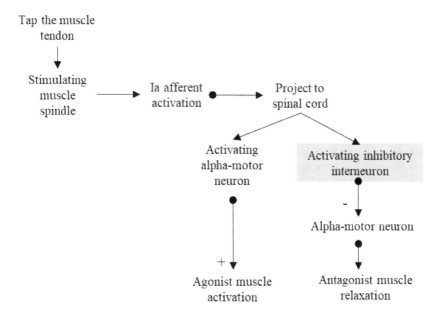

Figure 5.11. A flowchart shows an example of the process of a reciprocal inhibition reflex, which describes the relaxation of the antagonist muscles to accommodate contraction on the agonist muscle.

It involves several steps that occur in rapid succession:

1. Tap the muscle: The reflex is initiated by tapping the muscle that is to be contracted. This tap sends a sensory signal to the spinal cord through sensory neurons called type Ia fibers.
2. Activate alpha motor neuron: The sensory signal from the type Ia fibers synapses with alpha motor neurons in the spinal cord that innervate the same muscle that was tapped. This activation of the alpha motor neuron causes the muscle to contract.

3. Inhibitory interneuron: At the same time, the sensory signal from the type Ia fibers also synapses with an inhibitory interneuron in the spinal cord. This interneuron, in turn, sends an inhibitory signal to alpha motor neurons that innervate the antagonist muscle (i.e., the muscle that opposes the muscle that was tapped).
4. Antagonist muscle: The inhibition of the alpha motor neurons that innervate the antagonist muscle causes that muscle to relax. This relaxation allows the muscle that was tapped to contract without any interference from the antagonist muscle, resulting in smooth and coordinated movement.

Overall, the reciprocal inhibition reflex helps to ensure that the appropriate muscles are activated and inhibited during movements, allowing for efficient and coordinated motor control.

Reciprocal inhibition prevents muscles from working against each other when external loads are given. Abnormalities in the reciprocal inhibition reflex can also be seen in various neurological disorders, such as cerebral palsy, spinal cord injury, and multiple sclerosis. Treatment for these conditions may involve physical therapy or medications to help improve motor function and coordination.

Chapter 5: Spinal Cord Regulates Motor Function

Polysynaptic flexor reflex

The polysynaptic flexor reflex is often referred to as the *withdrawal reflex* because it results in the withdrawal of the affected limb from a noxious stimulus (Fig. 5.12). The terms "polysynaptic flexor reflex" and "withdrawal reflex" are often used interchangeably to describe this type of reflex.

During the withdrawal reflex, a noxious stimulus activates sensory receptors in the skin, muscles, or joints, which send signals to the spinal cord. These signals are then transmitted through a polysynaptic pathway involving interneurons within the spinal cord, which activate alpha motor neurons that innervate the flexor muscles of the affected limb. This causes the limb to be rapidly withdrawn from the noxious stimulus, helping to protect the limb from further injury or damage.

The withdrawal reflex is a type of polysynaptic reflex because it involves multiple synapses between different types of neurons within the spinal cord. This allows for a quick and automatic withdrawal response that helps to protect the body from harm.

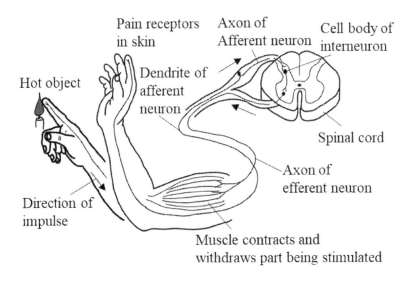

Figure 3. Polysynaptic flexor reflex. The figure shows an example of polysynaptic flexor reflex.

The process pathway for the withdrawal reflex can be described as follows:

1. Noxious stimulus: The withdrawal reflex is initiated by a noxious stimulus, such as a hot or painful stimulus, that activates sensory receptors in the skin, muscles, or joints.
2. Sensory afferent fiber: The activation of the sensory receptors sends a signal through a sensory afferent fiber, which carries the signal towards the spinal cord.
3. Spinal cord: The sensory signal enters the spinal cord and synapses with interneurons within the spinal cord.

Chapter 5: Spinal Cord Regulates Motor Function

4. Interneurons: The interneurons within the spinal cord process the sensory signal and send an output signal to activate alpha motor neurons.
5. Alpha motor neurons: The output signal from the interneurons activates alpha motor neurons that innervate the flexor muscles of the affected limb.
6. Muscle: The activation of the alpha motor neurons causes a rapid contraction of the flexor muscles, which results in the withdrawal of the affected limb from the noxious stimulus.

The withdrawal reflex is a protective reflex that helps to prevent further injury or damage to the affected limb. The reflex is an important part of the body's defense mechanism and allows for rapid adjustments in response to unexpected or painful stimuli.

Abnormalities in the withdrawal reflex can also be seen in various neurological disorders, such as spinal cord injury, multiple sclerosis, and stroke.

1. One example of an abnormality in the withdrawal reflex is hyperreflexia, which is an exaggerated or excessive reflex response. This can occur as a result of damage to the spinal cord or other parts of the nervous system, which can cause an increase in the excitability of the motor neurons. In hyperreflexia, the affected limb may exhibit a more pronounced withdrawal response to a noxious stimulus than is normally expected.

2. Another example of an abnormality in the withdrawal reflex is hyporeflexia, which is a reduced or absent reflex response. This can occur as a result of damage to the sensory or motor pathways involved in the reflex, which can impair the transmission of signals within the nervous system. In hyporeflexia, the affected limb may exhibit a weak or incomplete withdrawal response to a noxious stimulus.

Gag reflex

The gag reflex, also known as the pharyngeal reflex or laryngeal spasm, is a protective reflex that helps prevent choking and aspiration of foreign objects or fluids into the lungs. It is a reflex contraction of the muscles in the back of the throat, which occurs in response to stimulation of the soft palate, uvula, tonsils, or back of the tongue.

The gag reflex is activated by sensory receptors in the oropharynx, which send a signal through the sensory nerves to the brainstem. The signal is then processed and transmitted through the motor nerves to the muscles in the throat, causing a contraction of the pharyngeal muscles, closure of the glottis (opening to the trachea), and elevation of the larynx (voice box) to protect the airway.

The gag reflex can be elicited by a variety of stimuli, including medical instruments such as a tongue depressor or endoscope, as well as by unpleasant tastes or odors. In some individuals, the gag reflex may be more sensitive or easily triggered, while in others it may be less sensitive or absent. The absence of a gag reflex can indicate a neurological disorder or damage to the nerves involved in the reflex.

Crossed Extensor Reflex

The crossed extensor reflex is a type of neurological reflex that involves the extension of the opposite limb in response to a noxious stimulus, while simultaneously withdrawing the affected limb from the stimulus. This reflex is also known as the crossed-extension reflex (Fig. 5.13).

The crossed extensor reflex is polysynaptic, involving multiple neural connections in the spinal cord. It occurs when a noxious stimulus, such as a painful stimulus, is detected by sensory receptors in the skin, muscles, or joints. The signal from the sensory receptors is transmitted through a sensory afferent fiber to the spinal cord.

In the spinal cord, the signal is processed by interneurons that activate both the alpha motor neurons that innervate the flexor muscles of the affected limb and the alpha motor neurons that innervate the extensor muscles of the opposite limb. The activation of the flexor muscles of the affected limb causes the limb to be rapidly withdrawn from the noxious stimulus, while the activation of the extensor muscles of the opposite limb causes that limb to be extended and provide support for the body.

The crossed extensor reflex is important for maintaining balance and stability during movement. For example, if you step on a sharp object with your right foot, the crossed extensor reflex will cause your right leg to be withdrawn from the stimulus and your left leg to be extended to support your body weight, allowing you to maintain your balance and avoid falling.

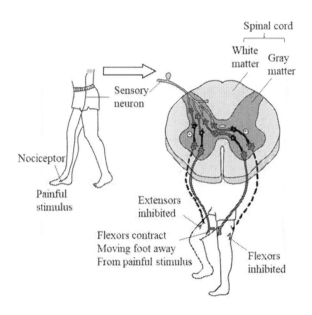

Figure 5.13. The figure shows the mechanism of a withdrawal reflex or crossed extensor reflex.

Chapter 5: Spinal Cord Regulates Motor Function

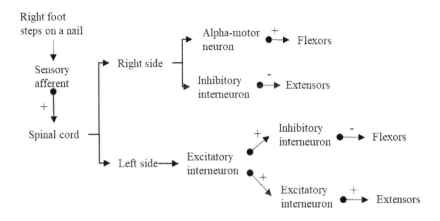

Figure 5.14. The flowchart explains the process of a crossed extensor reflex.

When the right foot steps on a nail, the pain signal travels to the spinal cord via sensory nerves. On the same side, the signal activates alpha-motor neurons, causing flexor muscle contraction. At the same time, the signal inhibits the extensors via inhibitory interneurons. On the opposite side (left side), there are two types of interneurons involved leading to an opposing reaction, inhibiting flexors and activating extensors. Therefore, this reflex is a contralateral reflex that allows the body to compensate on one side for a stimulus on the other.

There are a number of neurological disorders or injuries that can cause alterations or abnormalities in the crossed extensor reflex. Some examples include:

1. Spinal cord injury: Damage to the spinal cord can disrupt the transmission of signals between the sensory receptors and the

motor neurons involved in the crossed extensor reflex, leading to impaired or absent reflex responses.
2. Multiple sclerosis: This is a chronic autoimmune disorder that can cause damage to the myelin sheath that surrounds nerve fibers, leading to disruptions in neural signaling and impaired reflex responses.
3. Parkinson's disease: This is a progressive neurodegenerative disorder that can affect movement and coordination, including the ability to generate appropriate reflex responses.
4. Stroke: A stroke can cause damage to the brain or spinal cord, leading to impaired reflex responses and difficulty with movement and coordination.
5. Traumatic brain injury: This is a type of injury that can result from a blow or jolt to the head, leading to a range of neurological symptoms, including altered reflex responses.

Treatment for these conditions may involve physical therapy, medications, or other interventions to help improve motor function and coordination, as well as manage other symptoms associated with the underlying disorder.

Generation of spinal motor programs for walking

The generation of spinal motor programs for walking involves complex neural circuits in the spinal cord that are capable of

Chapter 5: Spinal Cord Regulates Motor Function

generating rhythmic patterns of activity in the leg muscles, known as locomotor patterns. These circuits are responsible for coordinating the complex sequence of muscle activations that are required for walking.

The process of generating spinal motor programs for walking involves several steps:

1. Sensory input: Sensory feedback from the limbs, muscles, and joints provides critical information about the position and movement of the body during walking. This sensory input is transmitted through sensory afferent fibers to the spinal cord.
2. Central pattern generators (CPGs): The spinal cord contains specialized neural circuits known as central pattern generators, which are capable of generating rhythmic patterns of activity in the leg muscles. These circuits are capable of generating locomotor patterns even in the absence of sensory input or descending commands from the brain.
3. Interneurons: Interneurons in the spinal cord act as intermediaries between the sensory afferent fibers and the motor efferent fibers. These interneurons help to integrate sensory feedback with the output from the CPGs, generating coordinated muscle activations that are required for walking.
4. Descending commands from the brain: While the spinal cord is capable of generating locomotor patterns on its own, descending commands from the brain can modify or adjust

these patterns based on the specific demands of the task. These descending commands are transmitted through descending pathways from the brain to the spinal cord, and can modulate the activity of the CPGs and interneurons.

Together, these neural circuits and processes enable the generation of spinal motor programs for walking. The spinal cord is capable of generating rhythmic patterns of muscle activation that are required for walking, while also integrating sensory feedback and descending commands from the brain to ensure smooth and coordinated movement.

The generation of spinal motor programs for walking has important applications in both clinical and technological settings. Some examples include:

1. Rehabilitation: Understanding the neural mechanisms underlying walking can inform the development of rehabilitation strategies for individuals with gait disorders or spinal cord injuries. Rehabilitation programs can be designed to target specific components of the spinal motor programs involved in walking, such as sensory integration, CPG activity, or descending control, to help individuals regain or improve their ability to walk.
2. Prosthetics: Advances in robotics and engineering have led to the development of sophisticated prosthetic devices that can restore mobility to individuals with lower limb amputations or

Chapter 5: Spinal Cord Regulates Motor Function

other mobility impairments. The ability to generate spinal motor programs for walking is critical for the development of prosthetic devices that can replicate natural walking patterns.

3. Robotics: The generation of spinal motor programs for walking has also inspired the development of robotic systems that can replicate or augment human locomotion. These systems can be used in a variety of applications, such as search and rescue operations, disaster response, or military operations.

4. Neuroprosthetics: In addition to prosthetics, the ability to generate spinal motor programs for walking has important implications for the development of neuroprosthetic devices that can restore or enhance motor function. These devices can be used to treat a wide range of neurological disorders, including spinal cord injury, stroke, and Parkinson's disease.

Overall, the ability to generate spinal motor programs for walking is a critical component of human locomotion, with important implications for both clinical and technological applications.

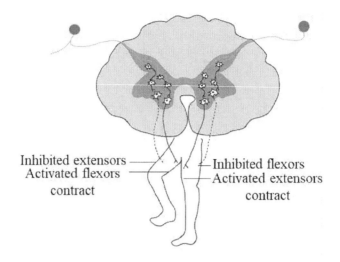

Figure 5.15. The central pattern generator. The picture shows the central pattern generator. The spinal cord generator plays a significant role in generating motor tasks. It has self-organizing biological neural circuits that produce rhythmic outputs without inputs.

What is an automated movement?

Automated movements such as the walking or running cycle, mastication, and respiration are generated by central pattern generators.

CPGs are located in the spinal cord or brainstem and are responsible for generating rhythmic patterns of muscle activation without the need for sensory feedback or descending commands from the brain. These circuits are capable of producing complex motor behaviors such as locomotion, respiration, and mastication, among others.

In the case of walking, CPGs in the spinal cord generate the basic pattern of muscle activation that underlies the walking cycle, but this activity can be modified by sensory feedback from the limbs and joints, as well as descending commands from the brain, to generate the specific muscle activations required for efficient and stable walking.

Similarly, the breathing cycle is generated by a network of CPGs located in the brainstem, which coordinate the activity of the muscles involved in respiration, including the diaphragm and intercostal muscles. This rhythmic pattern of muscle activation is modulated by inputs from respiratory centers in the brain, as well as feedback from respiratory muscles and chemoreceptors in the lungs and bloodstream.

Overall, CPGs are essential for generating the rhythmic, coordinated patterns of muscle activity that underlie many of the automated movements of the body. The study of CPGs has important implications for understanding the neural mechanisms underlying these behaviors, as well as for developing strategies to treat neurological disorders that affect these circuits.

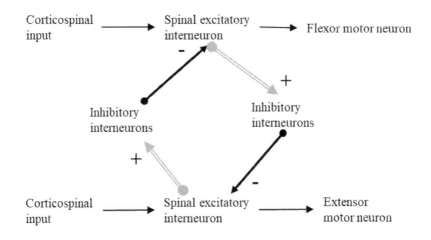

Figure 4. Oscillator model of the generation of spinal motor programs for walking.

This central pattern generator consists of two excitatory interneurons and two inhibitory neurons. The spinal cord's excitatory interneurons can generate spontaneous activity after losing the upper motor neurons. Therefore, this is an involuntary movement. One excitatory interneuron activates flexor motor neurons, while the other activates extensor motor neurons. Both excitatory interneurons send branch fibers to activate the inhibitory neurons (two inhibitory neurons). In turn, the inhibitory neurons can inhibit the excitatory interneuron.

There is ongoing debate among neuroscientists regarding the exact mechanism of central pattern generator (CPG) function. While there is general agreement that CPGs are responsible for

Chapter 5: Spinal Cord Regulates Motor Function

generating rhythmic patterns of motor output, the details of how these circuits work at the cellular and molecular levels are still the subject of active research.

There are several theoretical models of CPG function that have been proposed, including the oscillator model, the half-center model, and the chain model. Each of these models proposes a different mechanism for generating rhythmic motor output and has been supported by experimental evidence in different systems.

The oscillator model suggests that CPGs function like a biological oscillator, generating rhythmic motor output through the interplay of excitatory and inhibitory neurons. The half-center model proposes that CPGs are composed of two mutually inhibitory sub-networks that generate alternating periods of activation and inhibition. The chain model suggests that CPGs are composed of multiple interconnected modules, each of which contributes to the overall rhythmic output.

Recent advances in molecular biology and optogenetics have allowed researchers to probe the cellular and molecular mechanisms underlying CPG function in greater detail. For example, studies in the lamprey spinal cord have shown that the activation of specific classes of interneurons is sufficient to generate rhythmic motor output, supporting the oscillator model of CPG function.

Overall, while there is no single accepted model of CPG function, ongoing research is shedding new light on the cellular and molecular mechanisms that underlie these circuits and their role in generating automated movements.

What is nerve-induced plasticity of muscle fibers?

Nerve-induced plasticity of muscle fibers is the process by which muscle fibers can adapt and change their properties in response to alterations in their neural input. Specifically, changes in the pattern or frequency of nerve activity can induce changes in the phenotype of muscle fibers, including alterations in gene expression, metabolism, and contractile properties.

The process of nerve-induced plasticity is thought to be driven by a variety of cellular and molecular mechanisms. One key mechanism is the activation of transcription factors and other signaling molecules in response to changes in nerve activity. These molecules can alter the expression of genes involved in muscle development, metabolism, and contractile function, leading to changes in the properties of the muscle fibers.

Another key mechanism is the activation of proteolytic enzymes, which break down and remodel the structural proteins in muscle fibers. This process can lead to changes in the size and number of muscle fibers, as well as alterations in their contractile properties.

Chapter 5: Spinal Cord Regulates Motor Function

The process of nerve-induced plasticity can occur over a range of timescales, from rapid changes in gene expression and metabolic activity to more long-term changes in muscle structure and function. The degree and speed of nerve-induced plasticity can vary depending on a variety of factors, including the age and health of the individual, the specific muscle and nerve involved, and the nature and duration of the nerve input.

Overall, nerve-induced plasticity of muscle fibers is a complex process that plays an important role in the adaptation of muscles to changes in their neural input. Understanding this process is important for developing treatments for motor disorders and injuries, as well as for optimizing training programs for athletes and other individuals seeking to improve their motor performance.

Electromyography

Electromyography (EMG) is a diagnostic test that measures the electrical activity of muscles and the nerves that control them. EMG is used to evaluate and diagnose muscle and nerve disorders, including muscle weakness, muscle cramps, and muscle stiffness.

During an EMG test, a small needle electrode is inserted through the skin into a muscle. The electrode records the electrical activity of the muscle when it is at rest and when it is contracted. The results of the test can show whether the muscle is functioning properly, or whether there is a problem with the nerve supply to the muscle.

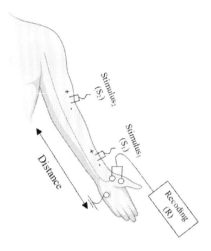

Figure 5.17. An electromyograph record of the thumb muscle controlled by a median nerve. It takes shorter time to travel from the stimulus 1 to the recording compared with the time to travel from the stimulus 2 to the recording.

EMG can be used to diagnose a variety of conditions, including carpal tunnel syndrome, neuropathy, and muscle diseases such as muscular dystrophy. It can also be used to monitor the progress of certain treatments, such as physical therapy or medication. EMG is usually performed by a specialist physician such as a neurologist or physiatrist who is trained in interpreting the results of the test.

Nerve conduction velocity test

A nerve conduction velocity (NCV) test is a diagnostic test that measures the speed at which electrical impulses travel through

Chapter 5: Spinal Cord Regulates Motor Function

nerves. The test is used to evaluate and diagnose nerve damage or dysfunction, which can be caused by a variety of conditions, including nerve injuries, neuropathies, and certain autoimmune disorders.

During an NCV test, small electrodes are placed on the skin over the nerve being tested. A small electrical impulse is then applied to the nerve, and the electrodes measure the speed at which the electrical signal travels through the nerve. The test may be repeated at different points along the nerve to determine if there is a problem with a specific area.

The results of an NCV test can provide information about the degree and location of nerve damage or dysfunction. For example, if the speed of the electrical impulse is slower than normal, this may indicate nerve damage or compression. The test can also help determine the extent of damage to the nerve, which can guide treatment decisions.

NCV tests are typically performed by a specialist physician such as a neurologist or physiatrist who is trained in interpreting the results of the test. The test is usually painless and only takes a few minutes to complete, although some people may experience mild discomfort from the electrical stimulation.

When do you use NCV test?

A nerve conduction velocity (NCV) test is typically used to evaluate and diagnose nerve damage or dysfunction. This test may be ordered by a doctor if a patient is experiencing symptoms such as tingling, numbness, weakness, or pain that may be related to nerve dysfunction.

NCV tests may be used to diagnose a variety of conditions that affect the nerves, including carpal tunnel syndrome, peripheral neuropathy, radiculopathy, and certain autoimmune disorders. The test can help identify the location and severity of nerve damage or compression, which can guide treatment decisions.

NCV tests may also be used to monitor the progress of a patient's condition or to evaluate the effectiveness of treatment. For example, if a patient with carpal tunnel syndrome undergoes surgery to relieve pressure on the median nerve, an NCV test may be used to confirm that the nerve conduction velocity has returned to normal.

Chapter 5: Spinal Cord Regulates Motor Function

SPINAL CORD INJURY

A spinal cord injury (SCI) is damage to the spinal cord that results in a loss of function or sensation. The spinal cord is a bundle of nerves that runs from the base of the brain down the back and carries messages between the brain and the rest of the body. An SCI can occur when the spinal cord is bruised, crushed, or severed, which can disrupt the communication between the brain and the body.

SCI can result in a range of physical and neurological impairments, depending on the location and severity of the injury. Some of the common effects of SCI include:

1. Paralysis or weakness of the limbs, trunk, or muscles used for breathing
2. Loss of sensation or altered sensation in the limbs, trunk, or other areas of the body
3. Loss of bladder and bowel control
4. Sexual dysfunction
5. Difficulty breathing, speaking, or swallowing
6. Chronic pain or spasms
7. Depression or other mental health issues

SCI can be caused by a variety of traumatic and non-traumatic events, including falls, motor vehicle accidents, sports injuries, and diseases such as cancer or multiple sclerosis.

The upper and lower motor injuries

An upper motor neuron (UMN) injury occurs when there is damage to the nerves that travel from the brain to the spinal cord. These nerves are responsible for initiating voluntary movement and maintaining muscle tone. When UMN injury occurs, there is a disruption in the signals from the brain to the spinal cord, which can result in muscle spasticity, increased muscle tone, and exaggerated reflexes. UMN injury typically occurs above the level of T12, which is the midpoint of the thoracic spine.

A lower motor neuron (LMN) injury occurs when there is damage to the nerves that travel from the spinal cord to the muscles. These nerves are responsible for activating muscles and initiating movement. When LMN injury occurs, there is a disruption in the signals from the spinal cord to the muscles, which can result in muscle weakness, flaccidity, and decreased reflexes. LMN injury typically occurs below the level of T12, which is the midpoint of the thoracic spine.

In general, UMN injuries are more common in SCI, especially in injuries that occur at or above the level of T12. This is because the nerves that travel from the brain to the spinal cord are more vulnerable to injury than the nerves that travel from the spinal cord to the muscles. However, the extent and severity of UMN and LMN injuries can vary widely depending on the location and type of injury, and each individual's response to SCI may be different.

Chapter 5: Spinal Cord Regulates Motor Function

Paraplegia

Paraplegia is a type of paralysis that affects the lower half of the body, including the legs and possibly parts of the trunk. It is caused by damage to the spinal cord, which disrupts the transmission of nerve signals between the brain and the lower limbs. The severity and extent of the paralysis may vary depending on the location and severity of the spinal cord injury.

Paraplegia can result from a variety of conditions, including traumatic injuries, such as those caused by motor vehicle accidents, falls, or sports injuries. Non-traumatic causes of paraplegia include infections, tumors, degenerative diseases, and genetic disorders.

Symptoms of paraplegia may include loss of sensation or movement in the legs, difficulty with bladder or bowel control, sexual dysfunction, and chronic pain. Individuals with paraplegia may also experience other medical complications, such as pressure sores, respiratory problems, and blood clots.

Treatment for paraplegia typically involves a multidisciplinary approach, including medical management, rehabilitation, and assistive devices such as wheelchairs or braces. Physical therapy and other forms of rehabilitation can help individuals with paraplegia to maintain or regain function and independence, while medications and other interventions may be used to manage pain, spasticity, and other complications.

Living with paraplegia can be challenging, but with appropriate treatment, rehabilitation, and support, many individuals with paraplegia are able to lead fulfilling and productive lives.

Quadriplegia

Quadriplegia, also known as tetraplegia, is a type of paralysis that affects all four limbs and the trunk. It is caused by damage to the spinal cord, which disrupts the transmission of nerve signals between the brain and the body. The severity and extent of the paralysis may vary depending on the location and severity of the spinal cord injury.

Quadriplegia can result from a variety of conditions, including traumatic injuries, such as those caused by motor vehicle accidents, falls, or sports injuries. Non-traumatic causes of quadriplegia include infections, tumors, degenerative diseases, and genetic disorders.

Symptoms of quadriplegia may include loss of sensation or movement in the arms, legs, and trunk, difficulty with bladder or bowel control, sexual dysfunction, and chronic pain. Individuals with quadriplegia may also experience other medical complications, such as pressure sores, respiratory problems, and blood clots.

Treatment for quadriplegia typically involves a multidisciplinary approach, including medical management, rehabilitation, and assistive devices such as wheelchairs or braces. Physical therapy and other forms of rehabilitation can help individuals with quadriplegia to maintain or regain function and independence, while medications and other interventions may be used to manage pain, spasticity, and other complications.

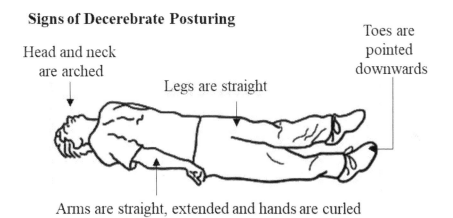

Figure 5. The signs of quadriplegia.

Spinal cord injury causes sensation Loss

Spinal cord injury (SCI) can result in loss of sensation, or altered sensation, in various parts of the body, depending on the location and severity of the injury. The spinal cord is responsible for transmitting sensory information from the body to the brain, and when it is damaged, this communication may be disrupted, resulting in sensory loss.

The extent and type of sensation loss will depend on the level of the injury. For example, injuries to the cervical (neck) region of the spinal cord may result in loss of sensation in the arms, legs, and torso, while injuries to the thoracic (chest) region may primarily affect sensation in the trunk and lower limbs.

Sensation loss may be partial or complete, and can include a range of symptoms such as numbness, tingling, burning, or the inability to feel hot or cold temperatures. In some cases, individuals may experience phantom sensations or pain in areas where sensation has been lost.

The loss of sensation can have significant implications for daily activities, including the ability to detect pain or injury, maintain proper body position, and perform self-care tasks. Rehabilitation and assistive devices such as braces, wheelchairs, and other mobility aids may be helpful in addressing these challenges and maximizing function.

Upper Motor Neuron Syndrome

Upper motor neuron syndrome (UMNS) is a neurological condition that affects the upper motor neurons, which are the nerve cells in the brain and spinal cord that control voluntary movements. UMNS can result from a variety of conditions that damage or impair these neurons, including stroke, multiple sclerosis, cerebral palsy, and spinal cord injury.

Symptoms of UMNS may include muscle weakness, spasticity (increased muscle tone), hyperreflexia (exaggerated reflexes), and abnormal muscle movements, such as clonus (rhythmic muscle contractions) or Babinski sign (the toes flex upward when the sole of the foot is stimulated). These symptoms may be more pronounced in the limbs on the side of the body opposite the affected area of the brain or spinal cord.

The specific symptoms of UMNS can vary depending on the location and extent of the neurological damage. In some cases, UMNS can lead to paralysis or complete loss of movement in the affected limbs, while in others, individuals may experience milder symptoms that primarily affect coordination or fine motor skills.

While UMNS can have significant implications for daily activities and quality of life, with appropriate treatment and management, many individuals with this condition are able to maintain a high level of function and independence.

Lower Motor Neuron Syndrome

Lower motor neuron syndrome (LMNS) is a neurological condition that affects the lower motor neurons, which are the nerve cells in the spinal cord that directly control voluntary movements of the muscles in the body. LMNS can be caused by a variety of conditions that damage or impair these neurons, including motor neuron disease, muscular dystrophy, and peripheral nerve injuries.

Symptoms of LMNS may include muscle weakness, atrophy (wasting) of the affected muscles, decreased muscle tone, and decreased or absent reflexes. The specific symptoms may depend on the location and extent of the neurological damage, as well as the underlying condition.

In contrast to UMNS, which is characterized by spasticity and hyperreflexia, LMNS is characterized by flaccidity and hyporeflexia. This means that the muscles affected by LMNS may be limp and unresponsive, rather than rigid and overactive.

While LMNS can have significant implications for daily activities and quality of life, with appropriate treatment and management, many individuals with this condition are able to maintain a high level of function and independence.

Pyramidal Signs

Pyramidal signs refer to a group of neurological signs and symptoms that are associated with dysfunction of the upper motor neurons in the brain and spinal cord. These signs include:

1. Spasticity: increased muscle tone or stiffness that affects the movement of limbs and makes them harder to move.
2. Hyperreflexia: exaggerated reflexes that can be elicited with tapping on tendons or other stimuli.
3. Clonus: rhythmic muscle contractions that occur in response to stretching or other stimuli.

Chapter 5: Spinal Cord Regulates Motor Function

4. Babinski sign: an abnormal reflex in which the big toe extends upward and the other toes fan out when the sole of the foot is stroked.

These signs can be indicative of a range of neurological conditions, including stroke, multiple sclerosis, cerebral palsy, and spinal cord injury. They are generally associated with upper motor neuron dysfunction, which can result in increased muscle tone and reflexes due to impaired inhibition of motor pathways.

While pyramidal signs can have significant implications for daily activities and quality of life, with appropriate treatment and management, many individuals with these signs are able to maintain a high level of function and independence. Treatment may include physical therapy, occupational therapy, and other rehabilitation interventions to address specific symptoms and improve mobility and function.

Pyramidal sign in respect to corticospinal and corticobulbar tracts

The corticospinal and corticobulbar tracts are two important pathways that transmit motor signals from the brain to the spinal cord and brainstem, respectively. The corticospinal tract originates in the motor cortex of the brain and descends through the brainstem and spinal cord, ultimately terminating in the lower motor neurons that control voluntary movement of the muscles in the body. The corticobulbar tract follows a similar pathway but terminates in the motor nuclei of the cranial nerves, which control movement of the muscles in the face, tongue, and throat.

Damage to the corticospinal or corticobulbar tracts can result in a range of neurological symptoms, including pyramidal signs. This is because these tracts play a critical role in the transmission of motor signals from the brain to the muscles of the body. Dysfunction or damage to these tracts can result in the increased muscle tone, hyperreflexia, clonus, and other symptoms associated with pyramidal signs.

In clinical practice, pyramidal signs are often used as an indicator of damage or dysfunction to the corticospinal or corticobulbar tracts. Depending on the underlying cause of the signs, treatment may involve a combination of physical therapy, occupational therapy, and other rehabilitation interventions to improve mobility and function, as well as medications or other interventions to manage spasticity and other related symptoms.

Similarity and differences of upper and lower motor neuron syndromes

Upper motor neuron syndrome	Lower motor neuron syndrome
Weakness or paralysis	Weakness or paralysis
Spasticity	Decreased or absent muscle tone (hypotonia or atonia)
Increased muscle tone (hypertonia)	Decreased or absent reflexes (Hyporeflexia or areflexia)
Over-responsive reflexes (hyperreflexia)	Involuntary muscle twitches (fasciculations)
Babinski sign positive	

Motor Neuron Disease

Motor neuron disease (MND) is a group of neurological disorders that affect the motor neurons, which are the nerve cells that control voluntary movement of the muscles in the body. MND is a progressive condition that results in the degeneration of these neurons, leading to muscle weakness, wasting, and eventually paralysis.

The most common form of MND is amyotrophic lateral sclerosis (ALS), which affects both upper and lower motor neurons and is characterized by muscle weakness, spasticity, and difficulty speaking, swallowing, and breathing. Other forms of MND include primary lateral sclerosis (PLS), which primarily affects upper motor neurons, and progressive muscular atrophy (PMA), which primarily affects lower motor neurons.

The exact cause of MND is not fully understood, but it is thought to involve a combination of genetic and environmental factors. There is currently no cure for MND, and treatment is focused on managing symptoms and maintaining quality of life. Treatment may include physical therapy, occupational therapy, and other rehabilitation interventions to improve mobility and function, as well as medications or other interventions to manage symptoms such as spasticity, pain, or respiratory problems. In some cases, assistive devices or other supportive care may also be necessary to address specific needs.

Are there MND genes?

Several genes have been associated with motor neuron disease (MND), although the exact genetic causes of the disease are not fully understood. The most common genetic mutation associated with MND is in the C9orf72 gene, which is found in up to 40% of familial ALS cases and 6% of sporadic ALS cases. Mutations in other genes, such as SOD1, TARDBP, FUS, and ANG, have also been linked to MND.

It's important to note that while mutations in these genes can increase the risk of developing MND, they are not the only factor involved in the disease. Environmental factors, such as exposure to toxins, may also play a role in the development of MND.

Genetic testing can be useful in diagnosing MND and identifying individuals who may be at increased risk of developing the disease. However, genetic testing is not always conclusive and may not identify all cases of MND.

Research into the genetic causes of MND is ongoing, and further advances in this area may lead to new treatments and interventions to prevent or slow the progression of the disease.

CHAPTER 6: BODY POSTURE, ARM REACHING, AND FINE MOVEMENT

Introduction

Body posture, arm reaching, and fine movement are all complex motor functions that involve multiple regions of the brain and various neural pathways.

1. Body posture refers to the alignment and orientation of the body in space, which is controlled by the postural control system. This system integrates sensory information from the eyes, inner ear, and muscles and joints to maintain balance and stability during standing, walking, and other activities. The postural control system involves various neural structures, including the cerebellum, basal ganglia, brainstem, and spinal cord.

2. Arm reaching involves the coordinated movement of the shoulder, elbow, wrist, and fingers to reach and grasp objects in the environment. This requires precise control of muscle activation and coordination, which is controlled by the motor

Chapter 6: Body Posture, Arm Reaching, and Fine Movement

cortex, basal ganglia, and cerebellum. The motor cortex initiates and plans the movement, while the basal ganglia and cerebellum refine the movement and adjust it based on feedback from sensory receptors.

3. Fine movement refers to small, precise movements of the fingers, hands, and other body parts, which are required for tasks such as writing, drawing, and playing musical instruments. Fine movement control is also mediated by the motor cortex, basal ganglia, and cerebellum, as well as specialized areas of the brain such as the somatosensory cortex, which processes sensory information from the fingers and hands. Fine movement control also requires the integration of visual and proprioceptive (body position) information to guide the movements.

HEAD AND NECK MOVEMENTS

Head and neck movements are important for many daily activities, including looking around, speaking, and chewing. Dysfunctions in the head and neck can result from a variety of causes, including injury, disease, and poor posture. Here are some common head and neck movements and dysfunctions:

1. Rotation: Rotation of the head and neck involves turning the head to the left or right. Dysfunction in rotation can result in limited range of motion, stiffness, or pain.

2. Flexion: Flexion of the head and neck involves bending the head forward. Dysfunction in flexion can result in neck pain, stiffness, or difficulty looking down.
3. Extension: Extension of the head and neck involves bending the head backward. Dysfunction in extension can result in neck pain, stiffness, or difficulty looking up.
4. Lateral Flexion: Lateral flexion of the head and neck involves bending the head to the side. Dysfunction in lateral flexion can result in limited range of motion, stiffness, or pain.
5. Swallowing: Swallowing involves a complex series of muscle movements in the head and neck. Dysfunctions in swallowing can result in difficulty swallowing, choking, or aspiration (inhalation of food or liquid into the lungs).
6. Speaking: Speaking involves movements of the tongue, lips, and vocal cords in the head and neck. Dysfunctions in speaking can result in difficulty speaking, hoarseness, or loss of voice.

Nerve supplies to the head and neck muscles

- Sternocleidomastoid (SCM) Muscle: The SCM muscle is innervated by the accessory nerve (cranial nerve XI).
- Trapezius Muscle: The upper portion of the trapezius muscle is innervated by the accessory nerve (cranial nerve XI), while the lower portion is innervated by the cervical spinal nerves (C3-C4).

- Platysma Muscle: The platysma muscle is innervated by the facial nerve (cranial nerve VII).
- Masseter Muscle: The masseter muscle is innervated by the mandibular nerve, which is a branch of the trigeminal nerve (cranial nerve V).
- Temporalis Muscle: The temporalis muscle is also innervated by the mandibular nerve, which is a branch of the trigeminal nerve (cranial nerve V).

It's important to note that these muscles are often innervated by multiple nerves, and that the nerve supply can vary slightly between individuals. Dysfunction of these muscles can result in pain, limited range of motion, and other symptoms.

Vestibulo-ocular reflex

The vestibulo-ocular reflex (VOR) is a reflex that allows us to maintain stable vision while our head is moving. It does so by coordinating eye movements with head movements to keep our visual field stable. When the head turns, the VOR generates an equal and opposite movement of the eyes in the opposite direction, which allows us to keep our gaze fixed on an object even as we move.

The VOR is initiated by the vestibular system in the inner ear, which detects changes in head movement and sends signals to the brainstem to generate the appropriate eye movements. The VOR is a critical reflex for maintaining balance and visual stability during movement.

Abnormalities in the VOR can result in a variety of symptoms, including vertigo, dizziness, and difficulty with balance and coordination. Causes of abnormalities in the VOR include:

- Vestibular Disorders: Disorders of the inner ear, such as vestibular neuritis or Meniere's disease, can result in abnormalities in the VOR.
- Traumatic Brain Injury: Head trauma can result in damage to the vestibular system and VOR abnormalities.
- Medications: Certain medications, such as antibiotics or chemotherapy drugs, can cause damage to the inner ear and affect the VOR.
- Neurological Disorders: Neurological conditions, such as multiple sclerosis or stroke, can affect the VOR and lead to abnormalities.
- Aging: As we age, our vestibular system may become less sensitive, leading to VOR abnormalities.

Treatment for VOR abnormalities depends on the underlying cause and severity of the condition. Physical therapy, medications, and lifestyle changes may be recommended to improve symptoms and prevent further damage.

Chapter 6: Body Posture, Arm Reaching, and Fine Movement

Cervicocollic reflex

The cervicocollic reflex is a reflexive response of the *neck muscles to head movements*. Specifically, it is a reflex that occurs when the muscles in the neck respond to movements of the head, which can involve tilting, rotating, or flexing the head.

This reflex involves sensory input from the cervical spine, which is transmitted to the brainstem and then back to the neck muscles via the motor system. The reflex helps to stabilize the head and maintain balance during movement, especially during rapid or unexpected movements.

The cervicocollic reflex maintains proper posture and preventing injury to the neck muscles and spine. It is also involved in the coordination of movements between the head and body, such as during sports activities or other physical tasks.

Overall, the motor control of head and neck muscles is complex and involves multiple neural pathways and feedback mechanisms. This complexity allows for precise and coordinated movements of the head and neck, which are essential for many activities of daily living.

Cranial nerves control head muscles

There are several cranial nerves that are involved in controlling the muscles of the head, including the face, eyes, tongue, and neck. Here's a brief overview of these cranial nerves and their functions:

- Cranial nerve III (oculomotor nerve): This nerve controls the movement of the eyelid, as well as the muscles that control the size of the pupil and the shape of the lens in the eye.
- Cranial nerve IV (trochlear nerve): This nerve controls the movement of the superior oblique muscle of the eye, which helps to move the eye downward and outward.
- Cranial nerve V (trigeminal nerve): This nerve has both sensory and motor functions and controls the muscles of mastication (chewing), as well as the muscles that control facial expression.
- Cranial nerve VI (abducens nerve): This nerve controls the movement of the lateral rectus muscle of the eye, which helps to move the eye outward.
- Cranial nerve VII (facial nerve): This nerve controls the muscles of facial expression, as well as the salivary glands and tear ducts.
- Cranial nerve IX (glossopharyngeal nerve): This nerve controls the muscles involved in swallowing, as well as the salivary glands.
- Cranial nerve X (vagus nerve): This nerve controls the muscles involved in speech and swallowing, as well as the muscles that control the heart, lungs, and digestive system.
- Cranial nerve XI (accessory nerve): This nerve controls the sternocleidomastoid and trapezius muscles in the neck, which are involved in head and neck movements.
- Cranial nerve XII (hypoglossal nerve): This nerve controls the muscles of the tongue, which are involved in speech and swallowing.

Chapter 6: Body Posture, Arm Reaching, and Fine Movement

Overall, the cranial nerves play a critical role in controlling the various muscles of the head and neck, allowing for precise and coordinated movements and functions.

Damage or dysfunction to these cranial nerves can result in motor dysfunction related to head and neck movements.

For example, damage to the facial nerve can cause weakness or paralysis of the facial muscles, which can affect the ability to make facial expressions or control movements of the head and neck.

In some cases, motor dysfunction related to the cranial nerves can be associated with conditions such as Bell's palsy, which is a type of facial paralysis caused by inflammation or compression of the facial nerve.

Similarly, damage to the accessory nerve can result in weakness or paralysis of the trapezius and sternocleidomastoid muscles, which can impair the ability to rotate or tilt the head or raise the shoulders.

Somatomotor cortex controls head and neck muscles

The cortex plays a critical role in controlling head and neck movement through its regulation of the cranial nuclei and other motor pathways.

When the motor cortex receives input from other regions of the brain, such as the sensory cortex and the cerebellum, it sends out motor commands via descending pathways, including the corticospinal tract, to the appropriate muscles. These motor commands control the timing, force, and direction of the movements of the head and neck muscles. The somatomotor cortex, which is a region of the cortex that controls voluntary movements, is particularly important in this regard.

However, dysfunction in the cortex can lead to problems with head and neck movement. For example, damage to the somatomotor cortex or other regions involved in controlling movement, such as the basal ganglia, can result in paralysis or weakness of the head and neck muscles. Similarly, disorders such as dystonia, which is a movement disorder characterized by involuntary muscle contractions, can also affect head and neck movement.

Other factors can also contribute to dysfunction in head and neck movement, including injury to the spinal cord or peripheral nerves that control the muscles, as well as certain diseases or conditions that affect the muscles themselves, such as myopathy or muscular dystrophy.

The cortical projection patterns to the cranial nuclei are mostly contralateral, meaning that the motor cortex of one hemisphere controls the muscles on the opposite side of the body.

However, there is an exception to this pattern for the facial nucleus, which is supplied by both hemispheres of the motor cortex. This bilateral supply provides redundancy and helps to ensure that

Chapter 6: Body Posture, Arm Reaching, and Fine Movement

damage to one side of the brain does not completely impair facial movements.

Regarding the frontalis muscle, it receives dual supply from both hemispheres of the motor cortex. This is because the muscle is involved in elevating the eyebrows, which is important for facial expressions, and has a unique innervation pattern compared to other facial muscles.

Overall, the somatomotor cortex is a crucial regulator of voluntary head movements and plays an essential role in ensuring the precise and coordinated control of the various muscles involved in these movements.

Head and neck muscle groups and motor dysfunction

The head and neck muscles are essential for proper functioning of the head, neck, and upper body. Dysfunction in these muscles can lead to a variety of conditions and symptoms, including pain, limited range of motion, and difficulty with daily activities. Some examples of head and neck muscle groups and associated dysfunction are:

- Neck Muscles: Dysfunction in the neck muscles can lead to neck pain, stiffness, and limited range of motion. This can be caused by poor posture, injury, or overuse.
- Facial Muscles: Dysfunction in the facial muscles can lead to a variety of conditions, such as Bell's palsy, which is a condition

that causes weakness or paralysis of the facial muscles on one side of the face.
- Mastication Muscles: Dysfunction in the mastication muscles can lead to temporomandibular joint (TMJ) disorder, which is a condition that causes pain and limited movement in the jaw.
- Extraocular Muscles: Dysfunction in the extraocular muscles can lead to strabismus, which is a condition that causes the eyes to point in different directions.
- Cranial Muscles: Dysfunction in the cranial muscles can lead to headaches, dizziness, and balance problems.
- Scalp Muscles: Dysfunction in the scalp muscles can lead to tension headaches and migraines.

Treatment for dysfunction in head and neck muscle groups depends on the underlying cause and may include physical therapy, medication, or surgery. Maintaining good posture, avoiding overuse, and practicing relaxation techniques can also help prevent dysfunction in these muscles.

Upper motor neurons control the head and neck muscles

The upper motor neurons controlling the head and neck muscles are located in the primary motor cortex of the brain. These neurons send axons down through the corticospinal tract, which runs through the brainstem and spinal cord. Within the spinal cord, the

Chapter 6: Body Posture, Arm Reaching, and Fine Movement

corticospinal tract neurons synapse with lower motor neurons in the spinal cord, which in turn innervate the head and neck muscles.

The corticobulbar tract is another pathway through which the upper motor neurons in the primary motor cortex control the head and neck muscles. This tract runs from the primary motor cortex to the brainstem, where the corticobulbar neurons synapse with lower motor neurons in the cranial nerve nuclei. These lower motor neurons then innervate the muscles of the face, head, and neck.

Both the corticospinal and corticobulbar tracts are responsible for controlling voluntary movements of the head and neck muscles. Dysfunction in these pathways can lead to a variety of conditions, such as spasticity, weakness, or paralysis of the head and neck muscles. Treatment for these conditions may include physical therapy, medication, or surgery.

Lower motor neurons control the head and neck muscles

The lower motor neurons controlling the head and neck muscles are located in the spinal cord and cranial nerve nuclei in the brainstem. These lower motor neurons receive input from upper motor neurons in the primary motor cortex and brainstem, and then directly innervate the muscles of the head and neck.

In the spinal cord, the lower motor neurons that innervate the neck muscles are located in the cervical spinal segments. These lower motor neurons receive input from upper motor neurons in the primary motor cortex and brainstem, and then send axons out to innervate muscles such as the sternocleidomastoid and trapezius.

In the brainstem, the lower motor neurons that innervate the muscles of the face, head, and neck are located in the cranial nerve nuclei. These lower motor neurons receive input from upper motor neurons in the primary motor cortex and brainstem, and then send axons out through the cranial nerves to innervate muscles such as the facial muscles, tongue muscles, and extraocular muscles.

There are several brainstem nuclei that control the face, head, and neck muscles, each of which is associated with a specific cranial nerve. Here are some examples:

- Facial Nerve Nucleus: The facial nerve nucleus is located in the pons region of the brainstem and controls the muscles of facial expression, including those around the eyes, mouth, and forehead.
- Trigeminal Nucleus: The trigeminal nucleus is located in the pons and medulla oblongata and controls the muscles of mastication, as well as other sensory functions related to the face and mouth.
- Hypoglossal Nucleus: The hypoglossal nucleus is located in the medulla oblongata and controls the muscles of the tongue, which are important for speech, swallowing, and other functions.

Chapter 6: Body Posture, Arm Reaching, and Fine Movement

- Accessory Nucleus: The accessory nucleus is located in the upper cervical spinal cord and controls the muscles of the neck, including the sternocleidomastoid and trapezius muscles.

These brainstem nuclei receive input from upper motor neurons in the primary motor cortex and brainstem, and then send axons out through their respective cranial nerves to innervate the muscles of the face, head, and neck. Dysfunction in any of these nuclei or their associated cranial nerves can lead to a variety of conditions, such as weakness, paralysis, or involuntary movements. Treatment for these conditions may include physical therapy, medication, or surgery, depending on the underlying cause.

Vestibulospinal tract controls posture and head movements

The vestibulospinal tract is a pathway that originates in the vestibular nuclei of the brainstem and descends through the spinal cord to control postural and head movements. It plays an important role in stabilizing the head during movements of the body and helps to maintain balance.

Dysfunction in the vestibulospinal tract can lead to a variety of symptoms related to balance and posture, as well as abnormal movements of the head. For example:

- Vertigo: If the vestibular nuclei are damaged or malfunctioning, it can cause vertigo, which is a sensation of spinning or dizziness.
- Nystagmus: Nystagmus is a rhythmic, involuntary movement of the eyes that can occur as a result of dysfunction in the vestibular system.
- Ataxia: Ataxia is a lack of coordination or unsteadiness that can result from dysfunction in the vestibular system and vestibulospinal tract.
- Head tremors: Dysfunction in the vestibulospinal tract can also cause involuntary tremors or shaking of the head, which can interfere with vision, balance, and other activities.

Treatment for vestibulospinal tract dysfunction depends on the underlying cause, but may include medications, physical therapy, or surgery. Vestibular rehabilitation therapy can be effective for improving balance and reducing symptoms related to vestibulospinal tract dysfunction.

Descending tracts of the spinal cord regulate movements

The descending tracts of the spinal cord can be divided into two main pathways: the lateral pathway and the ventromedial pathway.

Chapter 6: Body Posture, Arm Reaching, and Fine Movement

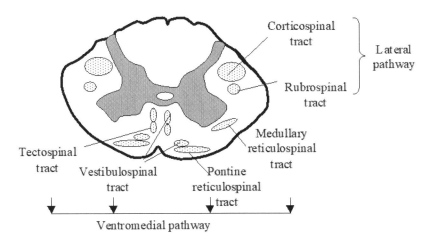

Figure 6.1. Descending tracts of the spinal cord.

The lateral pathway includes the corticospinal tract, which originates in the primary motor cortex and is involved in controlling voluntary movements of the distal muscles of the limbs. The rubrospinal tract also belongs to the lateral pathway and originates in the red nucleus of the midbrain. It plays a role in controlling limb movement and posture.

The ventromedial pathway includes the reticulospinal, vestibulospinal, and tectospinal tracts. These tracts are involved in controlling postural muscles and other involuntary movements. The reticulospinal tract originates in the reticular formation of the brainstem and is involved in modulating muscle tone and reflexes. The vestibulospinal tract originates in the vestibular nuclei of the brainstem and plays a role in maintaining balance and stabilizing head movements. The tectospinal tract originates in the superior colliculus of the midbrain and is involved in controlling movements of the head and neck in response to visual and auditory stimuli.

Overall, the descending tracts of the spinal cord are important for controlling voluntary and involuntary movements of the body, and dysfunction in these tracts can lead to a variety of motor impairments and disorders.

Tectospinal tract controls head movements

The tectospinal tract is a descending motor pathway that originates in the superior colliculus, a structure located in the midbrain. The primary function of the tectospinal tract is to control head and neck movements in response to *visual* stimuli.

When the eyes detect a visual stimulus, such as a moving object, the information is relayed to the superior colliculus in the midbrain. The superior colliculus then sends signals through the tectospinal tract to the motor neurons that control the head and neck muscles.

The tectospinal tract primarily controls the orientation of the head and neck in response to visual stimuli. For example, if you see a ball flying towards your head, the tectospinal tract will activate the appropriate head and neck muscles to move your head out of the way.

The tectospinal tract is particularly important for controlling rapid, reflexive movements of the head and neck in response to visual

Chapter 6: Body Posture, Arm Reaching, and Fine Movement

stimuli. This is known as the "orienting reflex," and it helps to protect the head and neck from potential harm.

Orienting reflex

The orienting reflex is a type of reflexive movement that occurs in response to a sudden or novel stimulus in the environment. It is an automatic response that helps us to quickly and accurately orient ourselves towards a potentially relevant stimulus. The orienting reflex is mediated by several different neural pathways, including the tectospinal tract.

If the stimulus is deemed relevant or potentially threatening, the orienting reflex is activated. This results in a series of rapid movements, including movements of the eyes, head, and body, that are designed to bring the sensory information into focus and allow us to better perceive and respond to the stimulus.

For example, if you are walking down the street and you suddenly hear a loud noise behind you, the orienting reflex will cause you to quickly turn your head and orient yourself towards the source of the sound. This allows you to better perceive and evaluate the potential threat and take appropriate action if necessary.

Therefore, the orienting reflex is an important component of our survival and adaptive behavior, as it allows us to quickly and accurately respond to changes in the environment that may require our attention or action.

How does the reticulospinal tract control head muscles?

The reticulospinal tract is a descending motor pathway that originates in the reticular formation of the brainstem and travels down the spinal cord. The reticulospinal tract is involved in the control of various muscles, including those that control the head.

The reticulospinal tract is divided into two pathways: the pontine reticulospinal tract (PRST) and the medullary reticulospinal tract (MRST). The PRST is involved in the control of extensor muscles, while the MRST is involved in the control of flexor muscles.

The reticulospinal tract can control head muscles through its connections with other motor pathways in the brainstem. For example, the reticulospinal tract can interact with the vestibulospinal tract, which is another descending motor pathway that controls head and neck movements in response to changes in balance and spatial orientation.

Chapter 6: Body Posture, Arm Reaching, and Fine Movement

The table shows the similarities and differences between the pontine and medullary reticulospinal tracts in the control of head muscles

Trait	Pontine Reticulospinal Tract (PRST)	Medullary Reticulospinal Tract (MRST)
Origin	Pontine reticular formation	Medullary reticular formation
Primary function	Control of extensor muscles	Control of flexor muscles
Connection to head muscles	Indirect, through other motor pathways (e.g., vestibulospinal tract)	Indirect, through other motor pathways (e.g., vestibulospinal tract)
Role in head movements	Can influence head movements as part of postural control and balance regulation	Can influence head movements as part of postural control and balance regulation
Interaction with other pathways	Can interact with vestibulospinal and tectospinal tracts in the brainstem	Can interact with vestibulospinal and tectospinal tracts in the brainstem
Lesion effects	Disruption of posture and balance regulation, leading to impaired head control	Disruption of posture and balance regulation, leading to impaired head control

In summary, both the pontine and medullary reticulospinal tracts can indirectly control head movements. The PRST primarily controls *extensor* muscles and can influence head movements as part of its broader function in regulating posture and balance, while the MRST primarily controls *flexor* muscles and may play a more direct role in the control of some head movements. Lesions affecting either pathway can lead to impaired head control as part of a disruption of posture and balance regulation.

BODY POSTURE AND BALANCE REGULATION

Trunk movements

Axial muscles are the muscles that are located in the trunk of the body, including the back, abdomen, and pelvis. They play an important role in supporting the body and maintaining posture, as well as in movements such as bending, twisting, and turning.

Function: Axial muscles are responsible for providing stability and mobility to the trunk of the body. They also help to maintain balance and control during movement. These muscles are important in breathing and other essential functions such as urination, defecation, and childbirth.

Here are some major axial muscles and their nerve innervations:

1. Erector Spine Muscles: The erector spine muscles are a group of muscles that run along the back from the sacrum to the skull. They help to maintain posture and extend the spine. The innervation of the erector spine muscles is by the dorsal rami of spinal nerves, which are branches of the spinal nerves that exit the spinal column.
2. Multifidus: The multifidus is a muscle that runs along the back of the spine. It helps to maintain posture and stabilize the spine. The innervation of the multifidus is by the dorsal rami of spinal nerves, which are branches of the spinal nerves that exit the spinal column.

Chapter 6: Body Posture, Arm Reaching, and Fine Movement

3. Diaphragm: The diaphragm is a dome-shaped muscle that separates the chest and abdominal cavities. It plays an important role in breathing. The innervation of the diaphragm is by the phrenic nerve, which originates from the spinal cord at the level of the third cervical vertebra.
4. Rectus Abdominis: The rectus abdominis is a muscle that runs vertically along the front of the abdomen. It helps to flex the spine and compress the abdominal contents. The innervation of the rectus abdominis is by the lower thoracic nerves, which are branches of the spinal nerves that exit the spinal column in the thoracic region.
5. Internal and External Obliques: The internal and external obliques are muscles that run diagonally along the sides of the abdomen. They help to rotate and flex the spine and compress the abdominal contents. The innervation of the internal and external obliques is by the lower thoracic nerves, which are branches of the spinal nerves that exit the spinal column in the thoracic region.

These are just a few examples of axial muscles and their nerve innervations. There are many other axial muscles in the body, and the innervation of each muscle can vary slightly depending on its location and function.

Movement: Axial muscles are involved in a wide range of movements, including flexion, extension, rotation, and lateral bending. These movements are important for activities such as standing up, sitting down, and turning the head.

Dysfunction: Dysfunction of axial muscles can lead to a range of problems, including poor posture, back pain, and difficulty breathing. Common conditions that affect the axial muscles include spinal cord injury, scoliosis, herniated discs, and muscular dystrophy. Physical therapy and exercises can help to improve the strength and flexibility of axial muscles, while medications and surgical interventions may be necessary in more severe cases.

The reflex loop maintains body posture and balance, which consists of information input and output, the peripheral nervous system, central integrative centers, and muscle responses.

Lateral corticospinal tract controls movements?

The lateral corticospinal tract (LCST) is a descending motor pathway that originates in the primary motor cortex and other cortical motor areas and descends through the brainstem and spinal cord. The LCST is responsible for the control of voluntary movements of the limbs, trunk, and distal musculature.

When an individual initiates a voluntary movement, such as reaching for an object, the decision to move is made in the motor cortex of the brain. The motor cortex sends signals through the LCST, which activates the lower motor neurons in the spinal cord

Chapter 6: Body Posture, Arm Reaching, and Fine Movement

that innervate the appropriate muscles. The LCST directly controls the movement of muscles on the *contralateral* (opposite) side of the body, meaning that the right LCST controls the left side of the body and vice versa.

The LCST plays a key role in the fine control of *skilled* movements, such as writing, playing a musical instrument, or typing on a keyboard. It can also help to generate forceful movements, such as lifting heavy objects or pushing open a door. In addition, the LCST can contribute to the control of posture and balance by activating the appropriate muscles to maintain an upright position.

Damage to the LCST can result in weakness or paralysis of the limbs on the opposite side of the body from the lesion. This is because the LCST is the main pathway for voluntary motor control of the contralateral limbs. Other symptoms of LCST damage can include spasticity (increased muscle tone), hyperreflexia (exaggerated reflex responses), and the Babinski sign (an abnormal reflex response in which the big toe extends upward when the sole of the foot is stimulated).

As the LCST descends through the brainstem, it is divided into several different subcomponents based on the location and function of the axons. These include:

1. The corticobulbar tract, which contains axons that control the muscles of the face, head, and neck. These axons terminate in

the cranial nerve nuclei in the brainstem, where they synapse with lower motor neurons that innervate the facial and cranial muscles.

2. The corticospinal tract, which contains axons that control the voluntary movements of the limbs, trunk, and distal musculature. These axons descend through the internal capsule and the brainstem, where they are further divided into the lateral and ventral corticospinal tracts.

3. The rubrospinal tract, which contains axons that originate in the red nucleus of the midbrain and descend through the spinal cord to control motor function. This pathway is involved in the control of limb movements and contributes to the control of posture and balance.

Overall, the LCST is a highly organized pathway that plays a critical role in the control of voluntary movement. Damage to the LCST can result in weakness or paralysis of the limbs on the opposite side of the body from the lesion, as well as other motor deficits.

The reflex loop maintains body posture

The reflex loop maintaining body posture has following components. The input from skin, muscles, and joints allows the central nervous system to interpret the body's position and make appropriate adjustments to maintain balance. The output from the

Chapter 6: Body Posture, Arm Reaching, and Fine Movement

central nervous system instructs muscle action to adjust body posture, which helps to prevent falls and other injuries.

The structures in the central nervous system mentioned, such as the vestibular nucleus, medulla oblongata, colliculi, cerebellum, and spinal cord, all play important roles in maintaining body posture and balance. The vestibular nucleus, for example, helps to detect head movements and orientation in space, while the cerebellum coordinates movements and helps to maintain balance.

Peripheral nerves are also important for maintaining body posture and balance. Any lesions on peripheral nerves can affect the transmission of information from peripheral organs to the central nervous system and from the central nervous system to the muscles, which can lead to problems with balance and posture.

Overall, the reflex loop and the various structures in the central nervous system, as well as the peripheral nerves, all work together to maintain body posture and balance during exercise and everyday activities. As an exercise physiologist, it's important to understand how these systems work and how to optimize them to help clients achieve their fitness goals while minimizing the risk of injury. Here are two examples of conditions that can commonly cause abnormalities in body posture:

1. Scoliosis: Scoliosis is a medical condition in which the spine curves to the side, leading to an abnormal posture. This condition can be caused by a variety of factors, including genetics, poor posture, or neuromuscular conditions. Scoliosis

can result in a range of symptoms, including back pain, uneven shoulders or hips, and difficulty standing or walking.

2. Parkinson's disease: Parkinson's disease is a progressive neurological disorder that affects movement and coordination. It is caused by the gradual degeneration of dopamine-producing neurons in the brain. Parkinson's disease can lead to a variety of symptoms, including tremors, stiffness, and difficulty with balance and posture. People with Parkinson's disease may develop a stooped posture or have difficulty standing up straight.

Other conditions, such as arthritis, stroke, or spinal cord injuries, can also lead to postural abnormalities. It's important to consult with a healthcare professional if you are experiencing any changes in your posture, as early intervention can often help to prevent further complications.

The reflex loop maintains body balance

This neural circuit allows for rapid and automatic responses to changes in the environment that may cause instability, such as sudden movements or uneven surfaces. The reflex loop is a neural circuit that involves a sensory receptor, afferent neurons, interneurons, and efferent neurons. In the context of maintaining body balance, the reflex loop works in the following way:

Chapter 6: Body Posture, Arm Reaching, and Fine Movement

1. A sensory receptor detects a change in the environment that may cause instability, such as a shift in body position or a sudden movement.
2. The sensory information is transmitted via afferent neurons to the spinal cord.
3. In the spinal cord, interneurons process the sensory information and send signals to efferent neurons that control muscles involved in maintaining balance.
4. The efferent neurons then send signals to the muscles, causing them to contract or relax, which helps to maintain or restore balance.

This process occurs rapidly and automatically, without conscious effort. It is essential in preventing falls and maintaining stability during everyday activities such as walking, standing, or reaching for an object.

However, it is important to note that the reflex loop is not the only mechanism involved in maintaining body balance.

The somatosensory, visual, and vestibular inputs also play a crucial role in regulating body balance.

1. The ankle region plays a critical role in somatosensory input. The superficial sensation derived from the skin around the ankle and the deep sensation derived from the ankle's muscles, tendons, and joints provide information about the body's

position and movement. This information helps the brain make adjustments to maintain body posture and balance.

2. Visual input provides the brain with information about the three dimensions of space position, which helps it instruct the body to adjust its posture and balance accordingly. Visual information also assists in determining the accuracy, magnitude, and movement time based on environmental conditions and changes.

3. The vestibular input plays a crucial role in sensing body movement in various directions, including up and down, linear acceleration and deceleration, and rotation. This information helps the brain make adjustments to maintain body posture and balance.

It is important to note that the somatosensory input is the most crucial, followed by visual input and vestibular inputs. Any abnormality in any of these three components can reduce the efficiency of regulation, making it difficult to maintain body posture and balance.

As an exercise physiologist, understanding the significance of afferent inputs is essential to design effective exercise programs to improve posture and balance. Exercises that target the ankle region, visual perception, and vestibular system can be included in the exercise program to improve afferent input regulation and maintain body posture and balance.

Chapter 6: Body Posture, Arm Reaching, and Fine Movement

Clinical examination of three input integrity for body balance control

The examination can be performed to evaluate the integrity of the inputs for maintaining body posture and balance. The outcomes of the assessments can assist in the differential diagnosis of diseases. As mentioned above, all three components (somatosensory, visual, and vestibular) contribute to maintaining body posture and balance. The test is based on removing or disturbing two elements from the total. The afferent input examined is normal if the subject can still maintain body posture and balance, as detailed below.

1. Examining Somatosensory (Ankle) Input: The subject is asked to close their eyes and put their head in a moving box. If the subject can still maintain their body balance, this indicates that the subject has normal somatosensory (ankle) input.
2. Examining Visual Input: The subject is asked to stand on a moveable platform and put their head in a moving box. If the subject can still maintain their body balance, the subject has normal visual input relating to balance.
3. Examining Vestibular Input: An examiner asks subjects to close their eyes and keep the platform under their feet in rotation (or sit). If the person can still maintain the balance, the person has normal vestibular input relating to body balance.

Three Steps of Rescue Reactions

The rescue reaction is the process by which the body regains balance after being subjected to an external force. This can happen, for example, when someone suddenly pushes you and you have to adjust your body to regain balance. There are three main steps to this process:

1. Stepping: This involves foot movements and is triggered by somatosensory input from the ankle region. This input is sent to the spinal cord via the spinal nerve, which activates a movement response. The reflex helps to catch the moving center of gravity, and ankle stiffness is a sign of this response.

2. Sweeping: This is a more complex reaction that requires a greater number of body movements. It involves the activation and coordination of both proximal and distal muscle reactions, with visual input playing a critical role in maintaining balance.

3. Protective reaction: This involves the activation of axial muscles, or trunk muscles, and is triggered by vestibular input. The response helps to protect the head from injury after a fall.

While somatosensory input from the ankle region is the most important factor in maintaining balance, visual and vestibular inputs also play a role. Ankle stiffness decreases as visual input is removed, and it decreases further when both visual and vestibular inputs are removed.

Chapter 6: Body Posture, Arm Reaching, and Fine Movement

Vestibular System regulates body balance

The vestibular system is an essential component in regulating body balance. It is a sensory system in the inner ear that provides information about the body's position and movement in space. The vestibular system works in conjunction with the visual and somatosensory systems to help maintain balance and stability. If the vestibular system is damaged or impaired, it can lead to problems with balance and coordination, which can impact a person's ability to perform daily activities and even lead to falls. Therefore, it is important to maintain the health of the vestibular system through regular exercise and other lifestyle habits.

Here are three common abnormalities related to the vestibular system:

1. Vertigo: Vertigo is a sensation of dizziness or spinning, even when you're not moving. It often occurs as a result of an issue in the inner ear, which can affect the vestibular system. The most common cause of vertigo is benign paroxysmal positional vertigo (BPPV), which occurs when small calcium crystals in the inner ear become dislodged and move into the ear canal.

2. Meniere's disease: Meniere's disease is a condition that affects the inner ear and can cause vertigo, tinnitus (ringing in the ears), hearing loss, and a feeling of fullness in the ear. It's thought to occur when there is a buildup of fluid in the inner ear, which affects the function of the vestibular system.

3. Vestibular neuritis: Vestibular neuritis is a condition that occurs when the vestibular nerve becomes inflamed, leading to vertigo, dizziness, and problems with balance. It can be caused by a viral infection or other factors that lead to inflammation in the inner ear.

Anatomical structure and function of vestibular system

The vestibular system, which is composed of the vestibule and semicircular canals, plays a crucial role in maintaining body posture and balance.

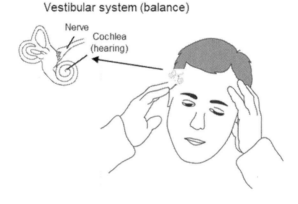

Figure 6.2. The vestibular system for balance regulations.

Vestibule: The vestibule, located between the semicircular canals and cochlear vestibule in the inner ear, consists of the saccule and utricle (Fig. 6.2). These structures sense body movement related to gravity and linear motion. The saccule contains the maculae, hair cells, and otoconia, which sense acceleration in the line of gravity. The utricle also has maculae that sense body movement and linear acceleration. The sensory cells in the saccule and utricle can convert mechanical signals generated by otoconia into electrical impulses, which are transmitted via the vestibular nerve to the brainstem. The vestibular nerve has cell bodies located within the inner ear, and the sensory information is processed in a topographic organization in the vestibular nucleus of the brainstem. The lateral vestibular nucleus processes information related to gravity and linear movement, while the medial vestibular nucleus processes information related to rotation. The output of the vestibular system regulates muscle activity in the head, neck, and shoulder regions, maintaining proper head position and protecting against injury.

Semicircular Canals: The three semicircular canals are C-shaped structures that sense head rotation in all three dimensions of body position. Each canal has an enlarged ampulla containing sensory receptors for head movement sensation. The anterior semicircular canal senses head movement anteriorly and posteriorly (like nodding "yes"). The lateral semicircular canal senses head movement horizontally (like shaking "no"). The posterior semicircular canal senses head movement medially and laterally (like tilting the head).

Common vestibular system abnormalities include benign paroxysmal positional vertigo (BPPV), Meniere's disease, and vestibular neuritis. BPPV occurs when otoconia become dislodged and move into the semicircular canals, causing brief episodes of vertigo. Meniere's disease is a disorder of the inner ear that causes episodes of vertigo, hearing loss, and tinnitus. Vestibular neuritis is an inflammation of the vestibular nerve that can cause severe dizziness and imbalance.

Three reactions for maintaining balance and orientation in space:

1. Righting reaction: This is a reflexive response that helps the body maintain its proper orientation in space. It is initiated by signals from the vestibular system in the inner ear, which helps the body sense changes in head position and movement. When the body detects a change in position or movement, the righting reaction is triggered, causing the head and body to move in such a way as to keep the body properly aligned with the vertical axis.

2. Placing reaction: This is another reflexive response that helps the body maintain balance and positioning in space. It is triggered by signals from the proprioceptive system, which helps the body sense the position and movement of its limbs and joints. When the body detects that a limb is in contact with a surface, the placing reaction is triggered, causing the limb to adjust its position and pressure to maintain balance.

3. Equilibrium reaction: This is a complex set of reflexes and movements that work together to maintain whole-body

Chapter 6: Body Posture, Arm Reaching, and Fine Movement

balance and stability. It involves the coordination of sensory input from the vestibular, proprioceptive, and visual systems, as well as the activation of specific muscle groups to maintain the body's center of gravity over its base of support.

All three of these reactions are important for maintaining balance and orientation in space, and they are all regulated by different parts of the nervous system, including the vestibular system, proprioceptive system, and cerebellum.

Imbalance with Sensory Ataxia

Imbalance with sensory ataxia is a common symptom seen in individuals with this condition. Sensory ataxia is a type of ataxia that results from damage to the sensory nerve pathways that carry information from the limbs and trunk to the brain. This can lead to a loss of coordination and balance, making it difficult to stand and walk properly.

Imbalance with sensory ataxia is often worse when visual feedback is removed, such as when the eyes are closed. This is because individuals with sensory ataxia rely heavily on visual cues to maintain their balance and orientation in space. Without visual feedback, their brain has difficulty processing information about the position and movement of their limbs, leading to increased postural sway and instability.

The causes of sensory ataxia can vary, and may include vitamin deficiencies, peripheral neuropathy, spinal cord injury, or other neurological conditions. Treatment for sensory ataxia may involve addressing the underlying cause of the condition, as well as physical therapy and balance exercises to improve coordination and balance. In some cases, assistive devices such as canes or walkers may be helpful in improving mobility and reducing the risk of falls.

Two examples of conditions that commonly cause imbalance with sensory ataxia are peripheral neuropathy and vitamin B12 deficiency.

1. Peripheral neuropathy is a condition that affects the peripheral nerves, which are the nerves that transmit signals between the spinal cord and the rest of the body. Damage to these nerves can disrupt the transmission of sensory information from the limbs and trunk, leading to sensory ataxia and balance problems.
2. Vitamin B12 deficiency can also cause imbalance with sensory ataxia. Vitamin B12 is essential for the proper functioning of the nervous system, and a deficiency can lead to damage to the peripheral nerves or the spinal cord. This can result in sensory ataxia and other neurological symptoms, including numbness and tingling in the hands and feet.

Chapter 6: Body Posture, Arm Reaching, and Fine Movement

There are many other conditions that can cause imbalance with sensory ataxia, including spinal cord injuries, multiple sclerosis, and Parkinson's disease, among others. Proper diagnosis and treatment of the underlying condition is important for managing the symptoms of sensory ataxia and reducing the risk of falls and other complications.

Romberg sign

The Romberg sign is a clinical neurological test that assesses an individual's ability to maintain balance and posture with their eyes closed. It is used to evaluate the function of the dorsal columns of the spinal cord, which are important for proprioception (the sense of body position and movement) and balance (Fig. 6.3).

To perform the Romberg test, the individual is asked to stand with their feet together and their eyes open, while the examiner observes their posture and balance. Then, the individual is asked to close their eyes and stand in the same position for a short period of time, while the examiner observes their ability to maintain their balance and posture.

If the individual is able to maintain their balance and posture with their eyes closed, the test is considered negative for the Romberg sign. However, if the individual sways or loses their balance when their eyes are closed, the test is considered positive for the

Romberg sign, which may indicate sensory ataxia or other neurological conditions.

It is important to note that a positive Romberg sign alone is not diagnostic of a specific condition, and additional tests may be required.

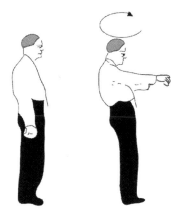

Figure 6.3. The figure shows sensory ataxia in Romberg's test when eye opening (A) and eye closure (B).

To examples of conditions that commonly show a positive Romberg sign are sensory ataxia and alcohol intoxication.

1. Sensory ataxia is a condition that results from damage to the sensory nerves or dorsal columns of the spinal cord, which are important for balance and proprioception. As a result, individuals with sensory ataxia may have difficulty maintaining their balance and posture when their eyes are closed, leading to a positive Romberg sign.

Chapter 6: Body Posture, Arm Reaching, and Fine Movement

2. Alcohol intoxication can also cause a positive Romberg sign. Alcohol affects the cerebellum, which is responsible for coordinating movement and balance. As a result, individuals who are intoxicated may have difficulty maintaining their balance and posture, especially when their eyes are closed, leading to a positive Romberg sign.

It is important to note that a positive Romberg sign is not diagnostic of a specific condition and should be considered in the context of other clinical findings and diagnostic tests. A neurological examination and additional tests may be needed to determine the underlying cause of the balance problems.

Cerebellar Ataxia

Cerebellar ataxia is a condition that results from damage to the cerebellum, which is the part of the brain responsible for coordinating movement and balance. As a result, individuals with cerebellar ataxia may have difficulty with fine motor coordination and maintaining balance, leading to unsteady and clumsy movements.

Patients with cerebellar ataxia typically exhibit difficulty with initiating and maintaining movements, which can lead to unsteady gait and difficulty with balance. This can be especially noticeable when starting a posture change, such as rising from a chair, and when walking. As you mentioned, patients may widen their base of support by walking with their legs widely separated to try to compensate for their imbalance.

Two examples of conditions that can commonly cause cerebellar ataxia:

1. Hereditary Ataxias: There are several types of hereditary ataxias, which are genetic disorders that affect the cerebellum and spinal cord. These can include Spinocerebellar Ataxia (SCA), Friedreich's Ataxia, and Ataxia-Telangiectasia, among others. Symptoms can vary depending on the specific type of hereditary ataxia, but common signs can include unsteady gait, difficulty with balance and coordination, tremors, and slurred speech.

2. Stroke: A stroke occurs when blood flow to the brain is interrupted, leading to brain damage. Cerebellar strokes can affect the cerebellum and cause cerebellar ataxia, along with other symptoms such as dizziness, nausea, and vomiting. Treatment for cerebellar strokes may involve medications to prevent further strokes, physical therapy to improve balance and coordination, and/or surgery to repair any underlying vascular problems.

Other potential causes of cerebellar ataxia can include head injuries, tumors, multiple sclerosis, and alcohol abuse, among others.

Decerebrate Posture

Chapter 6: Body Posture, Arm Reaching, and Fine Movement

Decerebrate posture, also known as decerebrate rigidity, is a type of abnormal posture that can occur as a result of damage to certain areas of the brainstem, such as the midbrain or pons. This posture is characterized by rigid extension of the arms and legs, with the arms pronated and extended at the elbows, and the legs extended and internally rotated. The posture is usually accompanied by hyperactive reflexes, and the patient may be unresponsive or in a coma.

Decerebrate posture is a serious neurological sign, indicating significant brainstem dysfunction, and can be caused by a variety of conditions such as traumatic brain injury, stroke, or brain tumors.

ARM REACHING

Arm reaching involves the coordinated activity of several muscle groups that work together to produce the desired movement trajectory and endpoint. The specific muscles involved can vary depending on the exact nature of the arm reaching movement and the position of the target object.

In general, the muscles involved in arm reaching can be grouped into three main categories:

1. Shoulder and upper arm muscles: These muscles are responsible for moving the arm into the desired position and orientation. The main muscles involved in this group include the deltoid, rotator cuff muscles (supraspinatus, infraspinatus,

teres minor, and subscapularis), and the biceps and triceps muscles.

2. Forearm muscles: These muscles are responsible for fine-tuning the movement and controlling the orientation and grip of the hand. The main muscles involved in this group include the flexor and extensor muscles of the wrist and fingers, such as the flexor carpi radialis, flexor carpi ulnaris, extensor carpi radialis, and extensor carpi ulnaris.

3. Scapular stabilizers: These muscles are responsible for stabilizing the scapula and maintaining proper alignment of the shoulder joint during arm movements. The main muscles involved in this group include the serratus anterior, rhomboids, and trapezius muscles.

The regulation of arm reaching includes:

1. Planning: The first step in arm reaching is the planning and selection of the appropriate movement. This involves several regions of the brain, including the frontal lobe, parietal lobe, and premotor cortex. These regions integrate information from the environment (e.g., the position of the target object) and the body (e.g., the current position of the arm) to generate a motor plan.

2. Initiation: Once the motor plan is generated, the motor cortex sends signals to the muscles involved in the movement to

Chapter 6: Body Posture, Arm Reaching, and Fine Movement

initiate the reaching motion. This signal is transmitted along the corticospinal tract, which connects the motor cortex to the spinal cord.

3. Coordination: As the arm begins to move, several brain regions and neural pathways work together to coordinate the motion and adjust the trajectory as needed. The cerebellum and basal ganglia play important roles in this process, providing feedback and adjusting the motor output to ensure smooth, accurate movement.

4. Feedback: Throughout the reaching movement, the brain receives continuous feedback from various sensory systems, including the visual, somatosensory, and vestibular systems. This feedback allows the brain to monitor the movement and make adjustments as needed.

FINE MOVEMENTS

Fine movements are typically performed by small muscles that allow for intricate control of movements. The following are examples of some of the muscles involved in fine movements:

1. Intrinsic hand muscles: These are the small muscles located within the hand, such as the lumbricals, interossei, and thenar and hypothenar muscles. These muscles allow for precise control of finger movements, such as typing, playing musical instruments, and manipulating small objects.

2. Eye muscles: The extraocular muscles are responsible for controlling eye movements, allowing for fine control of gaze and tracking of moving objects.

3. Facial muscles: The muscles of facial expression, such as the orbicularis oculi, orbicularis oris, and zygomaticus muscles, allow for fine control of facial movements and expressions.

4. Small muscles of the foot: The muscles of the foot that allow for fine control of movements include the lumbricals, interossei, and muscles that control the movements of the toes.

Overall, fine movements require precise control of small muscles, often in the hands, feet, face, or eyes, to perform intricate and delicate movements.

There are several diseases and conditions that can cause fine movement dysfunction, including:

1. Parkinson's disease: A progressive disorder that affects movement, causing tremors, stiffness, and difficulty with fine motor skills.

2. Multiple sclerosis: A condition that affects the central nervous system, including the brain and spinal cord, leading to difficulty with coordination and fine motor skills.

3. Cerebral palsy: A group of disorders that affect movement and muscle tone, often leading to difficulties with fine motor skills.

Chapter 6: Body Posture, Arm Reaching, and Fine Movement

4. Essential tremor: A neurological disorder that causes rhythmic shaking, particularly in the hands and arms, making it difficult to perform fine motor tasks.

5. Dystonia: A neurological movement disorder that causes involuntary muscle contractions and can lead to difficulty with fine motor skills.

CHAPTER 7: NEUROMUSCULAR JUNCTION DISEASES

NEUROMUSCULAR JUNCTION STRUCTURE

The neuromuscular junction (NMJ) is the point of contact between a motor neuron and a skeletal muscle fiber. It is a specialized synapse that allows for the transmission of signals from the motor neuron to the muscle fiber, which results in muscle contraction.

The neuromuscular junction (NMJ) is a specialized synapse that allows for the transmission of signals from a motor neuron to a skeletal muscle fiber. At the NMJ, the motor neuron releases a neurotransmitter called acetylcholine (ACh) into the synaptic cleft, which then binds to receptors on the muscle fiber's membrane called nicotinic acetylcholine receptors (nAChRs).

Binding of ACh to nAChRs on the muscle fiber's membrane leads to the opening of ion channels that allow for the influx of sodium ions, leading to depolarization of the muscle fiber's membrane. This

Chapter 7: Neuromuscular Junction Diseases

depolarization then triggers the release of calcium ions from the sarcoplasmic reticulum, which then initiates the process of muscle contraction.

The process of neuromuscular signaling and muscle contraction is crucial for motor control, allowing us to perform a wide range of movements and actions. Dysfunctions in the neuromuscular junction or in the signaling pathways involved in muscle contraction can lead to various motor control disorders, such as muscular dystrophy, myasthenia gravis, and spinal muscular atrophy.

Synaptic Cleft

The synaptic cleft is a gap between the motor end plate and the sole plate (Fig. 7.1).

The synaptic cleft, ~50 nm, is the space between the nerve terminal and the muscle membrane or sole plate. The nerve terminal releases acetylcholine into the synaptic cleft. The acetylcholine interacts with nicotinic acetylcholine receptors on the motor endplate.

The synaptic cleft has the enzyme acetylcholinesterase to catabolize acetylcholine; therefore, acetylcholine's effect on the post-synaptic receptors is short. The synaptic cleft can be divided into the primary and secondary synaptic cleft.

The primary synaptic cleft is a gap between the presynaptic and postsynaptic membranes. The secondary synaptic cleft is the invagination of the posterior synaptic membrane.

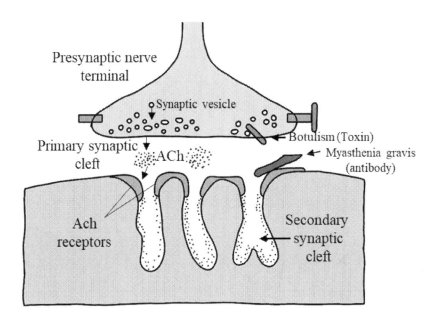

Figure 7.1. Structure of the neuromuscular junction. The figure shows the structure of the neuromuscular junction. The presynaptic nerve terminal releases acetylcholine (ACh) to the synaptic cleft. The figure indicates myasthenia gravis (antibody blocking nicotinic acetylcholine receptors), botulism (foodborne toxin, e.g., bacteria *clostridium botulinum*), and Lambert-Eaton syndrome (antibody attacks neuromuscular junction, an autoimmune disorder).

Chapter 7: Neuromuscular Junction Diseases

Motor End Plate

The motor end plate refers to the postsynaptic part of the neuromuscular junction, which is a portion of the muscle membrane, or sarcolemma. The muscle membrane protrudes into the muscle forming the junctional folds. The junctional folds have nicotinic acetylcholine receptors concentrated at the top. These receptors are acetylcholine-gated sodium ion channels. Acetylcholine and its receptors create endplate potential and generate action potential to the muscle membrane.

Transmission Pathway

Serial events occur during neurotransmissions from the neuromuscular junction. First, the motor nerve axon releases acetylcholine from nerve terminal vesicles into the synaptic cleft. Acetylcholine then binds to the acetylcholine receptor, located on the membrane of the muscle cell. Acetylcholine then induces an excitatory end plate action potential. As soon as the action potential is generated, acetylcholinesterase will hydrolyze acetylcholine. Because of this clearance mechanism, acetylcholine is removed from the synaptic cleft. The neuromuscular junction is reliable in function and fast-acting in response to stimulation.

TYPES OF ACETYLCHOLINE RECEPTORS

The table below shows nicotinic and muscarinic ACh-R in the control of muscle contraction:

	Nicotinic	**Muscarinic**
Muscle	Skeletal	Cardiac
Agonist	Nicotine	Muscarine
Derived from	Tobacco plant	Poisonous mushroom
Effects	Vomiting; large doses: Tremor and convulsion	Drop in heart rate and blood pressure
Antagonist	Curare	Atropine
Derived from	Arrow-tip poison (strychnos)	Belladonna plants
Effect	Paralysis of skeletal muscle	Large dose: Increases heart rate
Ion channel	Na^+	Ca^{2+}
Muscle membrane polarization	Rapid depolarization	Slow hyperpolarization

Chapter 7: Neuromuscular Junction Diseases

NEUROMUSCULAR JUNCTION DISEASE

Neuromuscular junction diseases are a group of disorders that affect the connection between motor neurons and skeletal muscles at the neuromuscular junction. These diseases can affect the transmission of signals between the motor neuron and the muscle fiber, leading to muscle weakness, fatigue, and other symptoms. Here are some examples of neuromuscular junction diseases:

1. Myasthenia gravis: This is an autoimmune disease that affects the nAChRs on the muscle fiber's membrane, leading to decreased sensitivity to ACh and muscle weakness. Symptoms can include drooping eyelids, difficulty swallowing, and weakness in the limbs.

2. Lambert-Eaton myasthenic syndrome (LEMS): This is a rare autoimmune disorder that affects the presynaptic voltage-gated calcium channels, leading to decreased release of ACh and muscle weakness. Symptoms can include muscle weakness, dry mouth, and difficulty walking.

3. Congenital myasthenic syndromes (CMS): This is a group of inherited disorders that affect the proteins involved in neuromuscular transmission, leading to muscle weakness and fatigue. Symptoms can vary depending on the specific type of CMS.

4. Botulism: This is a rare but serious condition caused by a bacterial toxin that blocks the release of ACh from the motor

neuron, leading to muscle paralysis. Symptoms can include difficulty swallowing, drooping eyelids, and respiratory failure.

5. Eaton-Lambert syndrome: This is a rare autoimmune disorder that attacks calcium channels on the muscle cells which can lead to muscle weakness.

Treatment for neuromuscular junction diseases may include medications that increase ACh levels or immunosuppressive therapy to reduce autoimmune activity.

What are the common symptoms of neuromuscular junction diseases?

The symptoms of neuromuscular junction diseases can vary depending on the specific disorder and its severity. However, some common symptoms of these disorders include:

1. Muscle weakness: This is a common symptom of neuromuscular junction diseases and can affect different muscle groups in the body. The weakness may be mild or severe and can progress over time.

2. Fatigue: Muscle fatigue is another common symptom of neuromuscular junction diseases. Patients may experience fatigue after minimal exertion or have difficulty sustaining physical activity for an extended period.

Chapter 7: Neuromuscular Junction Diseases

3. Diplopia (double vision): This symptom can occur in conditions like myasthenia gravis where the muscles that control eye movements are affected.

4. Difficulty speaking or swallowing: This is a common symptom in conditions like myasthenia gravis where the muscles involved in speaking and swallowing are affected.

5. Breathing difficulty: In some cases, neuromuscular junction diseases can lead to breathing difficulty and respiratory failure, which can be life-threatening.

6. Changes in muscle tone: Patients may experience changes in muscle tone, such as muscle stiffness or flaccidity.

7. Reduced reflexes: Reduced or absent reflexes may be observed in some neuromuscular junction diseases.

If you experience any of these symptoms, it is important to see a doctor for evaluation and diagnosis.

Myasthenia Gravis

Myasthenia gravis (MG) is a chronic autoimmune disorder that affects the neuromuscular junction, causing muscle weakness and fatigue. In MG, the immune system produces antibodies that attack the acetylcholine receptors (AChRs) on the muscle fibers, leading to a decrease in the number of functional AChRs and impaired neuromuscular transmission.

The hallmark symptom of MG is muscle weakness that worsens with activity and improves with rest. The muscle weakness typically affects the muscles of the eyes, face, throat, and limbs, and can lead to drooping of the eyelids, double vision, difficulty speaking or swallowing, and weakness in the arms and legs. Other symptoms of MG may include fatigue, shortness of breath, and changes in facial expression.

Diagnosis of MG typically involves a combination of clinical evaluation, blood tests to detect antibodies against AChRs, and electromyography (EMG) to assess muscle function. Treatment options for MG include medications that improve neuromuscular transmission, such as cholinesterase inhibitors and immunosuppressive agents, as well as plasmapheresis and intravenous immunoglobulin therapy to remove or block the harmful antibodies. In some cases, surgery to remove the thymus gland may also be considered. With appropriate treatment, many patients with MG can manage their symptoms and lead productive lives.

Chapter 7: Neuromuscular Junction Diseases

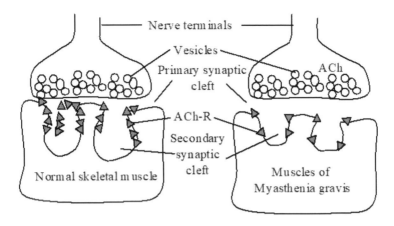

Figure 7.2. Number and density of acetylcholine receptors (ACh-R) in the normal (left) and myasthenia gravis (right).

The figure shows the number and density of acetylcholine receptors (ACh-R) in the normal (left) and myasthenia gravis (right). Usually, there is a dense accumulation of acetylcholine receptor binding sites on the sole plate of the skeletal muscle; however, there is reduced availability of ACh-R in myasthenia gravis.

Nerve Agents

Nerve agents are a class of chemical compounds that can affect the neuromuscular junction by interfering with the normal transmission of nerve impulses between motor neurons and muscle fibers. Nerve agents, such as sarin and VX, are designed to target and disrupt the activity of the enzyme acetylcholinesterase (AChE), which is responsible for breaking down the neurotransmitter acetylcholine (ACh) in the synaptic cleft.

By inhibiting AChE, nerve agents can cause an accumulation of ACh in the synaptic cleft, leading to overstimulation of the muscle fibers and ultimately, paralysis. This can result in a range of symptoms, including muscle twitching, weakness, respiratory distress, and seizures. In severe cases, nerve agent exposure can lead to respiratory failure and death.

Treatment for nerve agent exposure typically involves the administration of antidotes, such as atropine and pralidoxime, which can counteract the effects of the nerve agent by blocking the excess ACh and reactivating the inhibited AChE. Supportive care, such as mechanical ventilation, may also be necessary to manage respiratory distress and other complications. It is important to seek medical attention immediately if there is a suspicion of nerve agent exposure, as prompt treatment is critical to minimize the potential for long-term complications or death.

CHAPTER 8: SKELETAL MUSCLE

Skeletal muscles are the muscles that attach to the bones of the skeleton and are responsible for movement of the body. They are also known as striated muscles because their fibers have a striped appearance when viewed under a microscope.

Skeletal muscles are made up of thousands of long, thin cells called muscle fibers. These fibers contain multiple nuclei and are composed of bundles of myofibrils, which are composed of even smaller units called sarcomeres. Sarcomeres contain two types of protein filaments: actin and myosin. These filaments slide past each other when a muscle contracts, allowing the muscle to shorten and generate force.

Skeletal muscles are under voluntary control, meaning that they can be consciously controlled by the brain and nervous system. The contraction of skeletal muscles is initiated by the release of neurotransmitters, such as acetylcholine, from motor neurons that connect to the muscle fibers at the neuromuscular junction.

In addition to movement, skeletal muscles also play important roles in maintaining posture, generating heat to maintain body temperature, and protecting internal organs. Regular exercise and physical activity can help improve the strength and endurance of skeletal muscles, leading to improved overall health and wellness.

Size and shape: Skeletal muscles can vary greatly in size, shape, and arrangement depending on their location and function. Some muscles are composed of many small fibers, while others are made up of fewer, larger fibers. The shape and orientation of the fibers can also vary, with some muscles running parallel to the bone they are attached to, while others have a more oblique or diagonal arrangement.

Muscle fiber: Each muscle fiber is a single, multinucleated cell that is capable of contracting in response to a stimulus from a motor neuron. The arrangement of myofibrils within the muscle fiber gives it a striated appearance, and the sliding of actin and myosin filaments during muscle contraction produces force and movement.

Connective tissue: The connective tissue that surrounds and supports the muscle fibers plays an important role in transmitting force from the muscle to the tendon and bone. The blood vessels and nerves that supply the muscle provide the necessary nutrients and signals for muscle contraction and growth.

INTRODUCTION

Histology

Skeletal muscle histology refers to the microscopic structure of skeletal muscle tissue (Fig. 8.1). Under a microscope, skeletal muscle tissue appears striated, with alternating light and dark bands. These bands are caused by the arrangement of the contractile proteins actin and myosin within the muscle fibers.

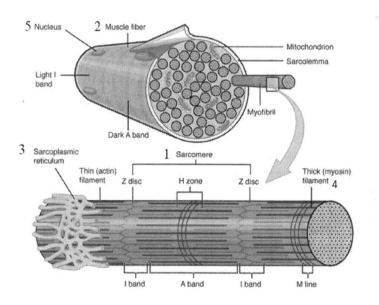

Figure 8.1. Structures of skeletal muscle.

The basic unit of muscle structure is the sarcomere, which is the part of the myofibril between two Z lines. Within the sarcomere, the thin filaments of actin are anchored at the Z line, while the thick filaments of myosin are located in the center of the sarcomere.

When a muscle contracts, the myosin filaments pull on the actin filaments, causing the sarcomeres to shorten and the muscle to contract.

Here's a summary of the key histological structures of skeletal muscle:

1. The A band (dark), I band (light), and Z band are structural elements of the sarcomere, the basic unit of muscle structure. Skeletal muscles are under voluntary control.

2. The sarcolemma is the plasma membrane that surrounds each muscle fiber.

3. Myofibrils are cylindrical structures located inside the muscle fibers. They are responsible for muscle contraction.

4. The sarcoplasmic reticulum is a network of tubules and vesicles that surround the myofibrils. It stores calcium ions (Ca^{2+}), which are released during muscle contraction.

5. T-tubules are invaginations of the sarcolemma that help to propagate the action potential into the interior of the muscle fiber. They also play a role in regulating the release of calcium ions from the sarcoplasmic reticulum.

6. Skeletal muscle fibers are multinucleated, with multiple nuclei located at the periphery of the cell. This allows for efficient protein synthesis and repair of damaged muscle tissue.

Skeletal muscle fibers are also surrounded by a layer of connective tissue called the endomysium, which contains capillaries, nerve fibers, and satellite cells. Several muscle fibers are bundled together into a fascicle, which is surrounded by a layer of connective tissue called the perimysium. The entire muscle is surrounded by another layer of connective tissue called the epimysium.

Skeletal muscle also contains two other types of protein filaments: titin and nebulin. Titin is the largest known protein and helps to anchor the myosin filaments in place. Nebulin is involved in regulating the length of the thin filaments and contributes to the elasticity of the muscle.

Skeletal muscle types

There are three main types of skeletal muscle in the human body:

1. Type I (Slow-Twitch or "Slow Oxidative"): These fibers contract slowly and are very resistant to fatigue, making them ideal for endurance activities. They contain high levels of myoglobin, which allows them to use oxygen efficiently. Examples include the muscles used for long-distance running and cycling.

2. Type IIa (Fast-Twitch or "Fast Oxidative-Glycolytic"): These fibers contract quickly and have a moderate resistance to fatigue. They rely on both aerobic and anaerobic metabolism to

produce energy. Examples include the muscles used for sprinting, swimming, and jumping.

3. Type IIb (Fast-Twitch or "Fast Glycolytic"): These fibers contract very quickly and are the most easily fatigued. They rely almost entirely on anaerobic metabolism to produce energy. Examples include the muscles used for powerlifting, throwing, and other explosive movements.

It's important to note that most skeletal muscles in the body are actually composed of a mixture of these three fiber types, with one type usually dominating depending on the muscle's function.

Muscles mainly made of type I muscles

There are several muscles in the body that are composed mainly of Type I muscle fibers, which are slow-twitch fibers that are adapted for endurance activities. These muscles are involved in activities that require sustained contractions over long periods of time, such as maintaining posture, running long distances, or performing activities that require sustained low-intensity effort. Examples of muscles that are predominantly Type I include:

1. Soleus: The soleus muscle, located in the calf, is mainly composed of Type I fibers and is responsible for plantar flexion of the foot.

2. Erector spinae: The erector spinae muscles, which run along the spine, are responsible for maintaining posture and are composed mainly of Type I fibers.

3. Diaphragm: The diaphragm, which is the primary muscle involved in breathing, is composed mainly of Type I fibers.

4. Slow-twitch muscles of the back: Many of the muscles in the back, such as the multifidus, rotatores, and semispinalis muscles, are composed mainly of Type I fibers and are involved in maintaining posture and stabilizing the spine.

5. Muscles of the neck: The muscles of the neck, such as the sternocleidomastoid and the trapezius, are composed mainly of Type I fibers and are involved in maintaining posture and movement of the head and neck.

Muscles mainly made of type II muscles

There are several muscles in the body that are composed mainly of Type II muscle fibers. These muscles are typically involved in activities that require short bursts of intense effort and power, such as sprinting, jumping, or weightlifting. Examples of muscles that are predominantly Type II include:

1. Biceps brachii: While the biceps contain a mixture of both Type I and Type II muscle fibers, they tend to have a higher proportion of Type II fibers, particularly Type IIa fibers.

2. Quadriceps femoris: The quadriceps are a group of four muscles located in the front of the thigh that are responsible for extending the knee joint. They contain a mixture of Type I and Type II fibers, but the vastus lateralis muscle, which is one of the four muscles in the quadriceps group, is known to have a higher proportion of Type II fibers.

3. Gastrocnemius: The gastrocnemius is a large muscle located in the back of the lower leg that is responsible for plantar flexing the foot and flexing the knee joint. It contains a mixture of both Type I and Type II fibers, but the proportion of Type II fibers is higher.

4. Deltoid: The deltoid is a large triangular muscle located on the shoulder that is responsible for arm abduction (i.e., lifting the arm away from the body). It contains a mixture of both Type I and Type II fibers, but the proportion of Type II fibers is higher in the anterior (front) portion of the muscle.

Type I and Type II muscle fibers differ in their nerve supply, with Type I fibers being innervated by smaller motor neurons and Type II fibers being innervated by larger motor neurons.

Molecular Basis of Muscle Contraction

The molecular basis of skeletal muscle contraction can be divided into three main stages: excitation-contraction coupling, sliding filament mechanism, and cross-bridge cycling.

Chapter 8: Skeletal muscle

1. Excitation-contraction coupling is the process by which an action potential (electrical signal) in the muscle fiber membrane (sarcolemma) triggers the release of calcium ions (Ca2+) from the sarcoplasmic reticulum (SR) within the muscle fiber. This release of Ca2+ causes the binding of Ca2+ to the regulatory protein troponin, which exposes the myosin-binding sites on actin, allowing the sliding filament mechanism to occur.
2. The sliding filament mechanism is the process by which the myosin heads on thick filaments bind to the actin molecules on thin filaments, forming cross-bridges. The myosin heads then undergo a conformational change, pulling the thin filaments towards the center of the sarcomere (the basic contractile unit of muscle). This process is powered by the hydrolysis of ATP to ADP and inorganic phosphate (Pi), which provides energy for the movement of the myosin heads.
3. Cross-bridge cycling is the process by which the myosin heads detach from actin, reposition themselves, and reattach to a new actin molecule, in order to continue the sliding filament mechanism. This process is regulated by the presence of Ca2+ ions, which activate the myosin-ATPase enzyme that hydrolyzes ATP and triggers the movement of the myosin heads.

Overall, the molecular basis of skeletal muscle contraction involves a complex interplay between various proteins and signaling pathways within muscle fibers, which enables the generation of force and movement.

Nutrition requirements for types I and type II muscles

There are some nutritional requirements that differ between Type I and Type II muscle fibers, as they have different metabolic characteristics and energy demands.

Type I muscle fibers have a high oxidative capacity and rely primarily on aerobic metabolism to produce energy. They also have a high concentration of mitochondria, which are responsible for producing energy in cells. As a result, Type I muscle fibers require a steady supply of oxygen and nutrients, such as glucose and fatty acids, to support their energy needs. Diets high in *complex carbohydrates* and *healthy fats* can be beneficial for Type I muscle fibers, as they provide a sustained source of energy for endurance activities. Additionally, consuming foods high in *antioxidants*, such as fruits and vegetables, can help protect Type I muscle fibers from oxidative damage during prolonged exercise.

Type II muscle fibers, on the other hand, have a lower oxidative capacity and rely more on anaerobic metabolism to produce energy. They also have a high concentration of glycogen, which is the storage form of glucose in the body. As a result, Type II muscle fibers require a readily available source of *glucose* to support their energy needs. Diets high in *simple carbohydrates*, such as sugars and white flour, can be beneficial for Type II muscle fibers, as they provide a quick source of energy for high-intensity activities.

Additionally, consuming foods high in *protein* can help support the growth and repair of Type II muscle fibers after exercise.

Overall, a well-rounded diet that includes a balance of complex carbohydrates, healthy fats, protein, and antioxidants can be beneficial for both Type I and Type II muscle fibers. Additionally, staying hydrated and consuming adequate electrolytes, such as sodium and potassium, can help support muscle function during exercise.

Exercises influence muscle fiber types

Yes, Type I and Type II muscle fibers respond differently to exercise, as they have different metabolic and structural characteristics.

Type I muscle fibers are adapted for endurance activities and have a high oxidative capacity. Endurance exercise, such as long-distance running or cycling, can increase the number and size of mitochondria in Type I muscle fibers, which improves their ability to produce energy through aerobic metabolism. Endurance exercise can also improve the capillary network surrounding Type I muscle fibers, which allows for increased delivery of oxygen and nutrients to the muscle. Overall, regular endurance exercise can lead to improvements in the endurance and fatigue resistance of Type I muscle fibers.

Type II muscle fibers, on the other hand, are adapted for high-intensity, short-duration activities and have a lower oxidative capacity. High-intensity exercise, such as weight lifting or sprinting, can increase the size and strength of Type II muscle fibers, as well as the amount of stored glycogen. High-intensity exercise can also improve the ability of Type II muscle fibers to produce energy through anaerobic metabolism, which allows for increased power and speed. Overall, regular high-intensity exercise can lead to improvements in the strength and power of Type II muscle fibers.

Neuron or muscle changes first when we age

The neural changes associated with aging can occur before the muscle changes. As people age, there is a gradual loss of motor neurons, particularly the larger and more powerful motor neurons that innervate the fast-twitch muscle fibers. This can lead to a reduction in muscle fiber size, strength, and power output.

In addition to changes in the number and function of motor neurons, aging can also lead to changes in the neuromuscular junction, the point where the motor neuron meets the muscle fiber. These changes can affect the ability of the motor neuron to stimulate the muscle fiber, which can further contribute to muscle weakness and atrophy.

Therefore, while the exact timeline of neural and muscle changes with aging can vary between individuals, it is generally thought that neural changes can occur before the muscle changes, particularly in the larger, more powerful muscles of the body. However, it is important to note that both neural and muscle changes can occur with aging and can contribute to the age-related decline in muscle function.

Muscle dysfunction

Muscle dysfunction refers to a condition where the muscles are not functioning properly. This can manifest in several ways, including weakness, fatigue, spasms, cramps, and pain. There are several underlying causes of muscle dysfunction, including:

1. Neurological disorders: Conditions such as multiple sclerosis, Parkinson's disease, and motor neuron disease can all cause muscle dysfunction.

2. Metabolic disorders: Disorders such as hypothyroidism, hyperthyroidism, and diabetes can affect muscle function.

3. Inflammatory conditions: Conditions such as polymyositis and dermatomyositis can cause muscle weakness and dysfunction.

4. Trauma: Traumatic injuries to the muscles, such as strains and sprains, can cause dysfunction.

5. Medications: Certain medications, such as statins used to lower cholesterol, can cause muscle dysfunction.

Treatment of muscle dysfunction depends on the underlying cause. In some cases, lifestyle changes such as exercise, stretching, and proper nutrition can help alleviate symptoms. In other cases, medications or other medical interventions may be necessary. It is important to consult with a healthcare professional for an accurate diagnosis and treatment plan.

MUSCLE WEAKNESS

Muscle weakness is a condition characterized by a decrease in the strength of one or more muscles in the body. Some common symptoms of muscle weakness include difficulty lifting or holding objects, trouble walking or climbing stairs, frequent falls, and fatigue. The muscle weakness can be caused by a variety of factors, including neurological disorders, muscular diseases, autoimmune disorders, hormonal imbalances, infections, and certain medications.

The following are the primary causes of muscle weakness:

Muscle weakness caused by upper motor neuron lesion

Muscle weakness caused by upper motor neurons is known as upper motor neuron syndrome. Upper motor neurons are nerve cells that originate in the brain and carry messages to the spinal cord, where they connect with lower motor neurons that control muscle movement. When upper motor neurons are damaged or impaired, it can lead to muscle weakness, spasticity (stiffness), and other neurological symptoms.

Some common causes of upper motor neuron syndrome include:

1. Stroke: A stroke can damage the upper motor neurons that control muscle movement, leading to muscle weakness and other symptoms.
2. Multiple sclerosis (MS): MS can cause damage to the upper motor neurons, leading to muscle weakness and other neurological symptoms.
3. Traumatic brain injury: Traumatic brain injury can damage the upper motor neurons, leading to muscle weakness and other neurological symptoms.
4. Spinal cord injury: Spinal cord injury can damage the upper motor neurons that control muscle movement, leading to muscle weakness and spasticity.
5. Amyotrophic lateral sclerosis (ALS): ALS is a progressive neurological disorder that can affect the upper motor neurons, leading to muscle weakness and other symptoms.
6. Cerebral palsy: Cerebral palsy is a neurological disorder that can cause damage to the upper motor neurons, leading to muscle weakness and spasticity.

Treatment for muscle weakness caused by upper motor neuron syndrome may include physical therapy, medication, or surgery, depending on the underlying cause and severity of symptoms. A healthcare professional should be consulted for evaluation and diagnosis.

Muscle weakness caused by lower motor neuron injury

Muscle weakness caused by lower motor neuron injury is known as lower motor neuron syndrome. Lower motor neurons are nerve cells that originate in the spinal cord and carry messages from the brain to the muscles. When lower motor neurons are damaged or impaired, it can lead to muscle weakness, atrophy (loss of muscle mass), and other neurological symptoms.

Some common causes of lower motor neuron syndrome include:

1. Spinal cord injury: Spinal cord injury can damage the lower motor neurons that control muscle movement, leading to muscle weakness and atrophy.
2. Peripheral neuropathy: Peripheral neuropathy is a condition in which the nerves that control muscle movement in the arms and legs are damaged, leading to muscle weakness, atrophy, and other symptoms.
3. Muscular dystrophy: Muscular dystrophy is a group of genetic disorders that can cause damage to the lower motor neurons, leading to muscle weakness and atrophy.
4. Polio: Polio is a viral infection that can damage the lower motor neurons, leading to muscle weakness and atrophy.
5. Amyotrophic lateral sclerosis (ALS): ALS is a progressive neurological disorder that can affect the lower motor neurons, leading to muscle weakness, atrophy, and other symptoms.

6. Guillain-Barre syndrome: Guillain-Barre syndrome is a rare neurological disorder that can cause damage to the lower motor neurons, leading to muscle weakness, atrophy, and paralysis.

Treatment for muscle weakness caused by lower motor neuron syndrome depends on the underlying cause and may include physical therapy, medication, or surgery. A healthcare professional should be consulted for evaluation and diagnosis.

Muscle weakness and myopathy

Muscle weakness can be a symptom of myopathy, which is a group of diseases that affect the muscles. Myopathy can be caused by a variety of factors, including genetic mutations, autoimmune disorders, infections, and exposure to certain toxins.

Symptoms: Myopathy can cause muscle weakness, as well as other symptoms such as muscle pain, stiffness, cramping, and fatigue. The specific symptoms and severity of myopathy depend on the underlying cause and the muscles affected.

Causes: Myopathic weakness can be due to damage within the motor unit that affects the muscle fibers or neuromuscular junctions. There is a decrease in the number of contractions of the muscle fibers activated with the motor unit. Many factors can damage muscle fibers, such as inflammatory, congenital, mitochondrial, and metabolic myopathy or muscular dystrophies.

The muscles can still contract but with less strength than normal muscles.

Diagnosis of myopathy typically involves a physical exam, blood tests, and imaging studies such as an electromyography (EMG) or a muscle biopsy. Treatment for myopathy depends on the underlying cause and may include medications, physical therapy, and lifestyle modifications.

Neurogenic muscle weakness

Neurogenic muscle weakness is a type of muscle weakness that is caused by damage or dysfunction of the nerves that control the muscles. This can occur due to a variety of neurological conditions, including:

1. Peripheral neuropathy: Peripheral neuropathy is a condition that affects the nerves outside of the brain and spinal cord, causing muscle weakness, numbness, and pain.
2. Spinal cord injury: Injury to the spinal cord can cause damage to the nerves that control the muscles, leading to muscle weakness and paralysis.
3. Multiple sclerosis: Multiple sclerosis is a neurological disorder that affects the central nervous system, causing muscle weakness, fatigue, and other symptoms.
4. Amyotrophic lateral sclerosis (ALS): ALS is a progressive neurological disorder that affects the motor neurons in the

brain and spinal cord, leading to muscle weakness, atrophy, and paralysis.

5. Guillain-Barre syndrome: Guillain-Barre syndrome is a rare disorder in which the immune system attacks the nerves, causing muscle weakness, paralysis, and other symptoms.

The symptoms of neurogenic muscle weakness depend on the underlying cause and the extent of nerve damage. Common symptoms include muscle weakness, atrophy, and twitching, as well as numbness, tingling, and pain.

The table shows the symptoms of three basic patterns of skeletal muscle weakness

	Upper motor neuron	Lower motor neuron	Myopathic
Atrophy	-	Severe	Mild
Fasciculation	-	Common	-
Tone	Spastic	Decreased	Normal/decreased
Distribution of weakness	Regional	Segmental/distal	Proximal
Tendon reflex	Hyperactive	Hypoactive/absent	Normal/hypoactive
Babinski's sign	Yes	No	No

(Based on Wilson, JD et al., [1991]. *Principles of Internal Medicine*, New York, McGraw-Hill Inc.)

MYOPATHY

Myopathies are a group of disorders that affect the muscles. These disorders can affect the structure, function, and metabolism of muscles. There are many types of myopathies, including genetic and acquired myopathies.

The most common symptoms of myopathy include muscle weakness, pain, cramps, fatigue, and difficulty standing, walking, or swallowing. The severity of symptoms can vary widely depending on the underlying cause and the specific type of myopathy.

Genetic myopathies are caused by inherited genetic mutations that affect muscle function. Some examples of genetic myopathies include:

1. Duchenne muscular dystrophy: A genetic disorder that affects muscle function and causes progressive muscle weakness and wasting.

2. Myotonic dystrophy: A genetic disorder that causes muscle weakness and wasting, as well as other symptoms such as heart problems and cognitive impairment.

3. Congenital myopathies: A group of genetic disorders that affect muscle function and cause muscle weakness and wasting from birth.

Acquired myopathies are caused by factors other than genetics, such as medications, infections, and autoimmune disorders. Some examples of acquired myopathies include:

1. Inflammatory myopathies: A group of autoimmune disorders that cause inflammation and damage to muscles, leading to muscle weakness and wasting.

2. Drug-induced myopathies: Certain medications, such as statins used to lower cholesterol, can cause muscle damage and weakness.

3. Metabolic myopathies: Disorders such as Pompe disease, which affect the metabolism of sugars in the body, can cause muscle weakness and wasting.

Duchenne Muscle Dystrophy

Duchenne muscular dystrophy (DMD) is a genetic disorder that causes progressive muscle weakness and degeneration. It is one of the most common forms of muscular dystrophy, affecting approximately 1 in every 3,500 to 5,000 male births.

MD is caused by mutations in the dystrophin gene, which codes for a protein called dystrophin that is important for maintaining the structure and function of muscle fibers. In individuals with DMD, the absence of dystrophin results in the progressive breakdown and loss of muscle tissue.

Symptoms of DMD typically begin in early childhood, with affected children exhibiting delayed motor milestones, such as walking and running. Other symptoms may include:

- Muscle weakness and atrophy, particularly in the legs and pelvis
- Difficulty standing up from a seated position or climbing stairs

- Gait abnormalities, such as walking on the toes or waddling
- Enlarged calf muscles (pseudohypertrophy)
- Contractures (permanent muscle tightening) in the joints
- Cardiomyopathy (heart muscle weakness) and respiratory problems in later stages of the disease

Clinical features: The symptoms start at an early stage of childhood (about two years of age). The patients have weak pelvic and shoulder girdle muscles and a waddling gait. Gower's sign is present. The symptoms gradually become severe. Patients often have to be in a wheelchair before age twelve.

Gower's sign: Gower's sign occurs when a patient encounters difficulty rising from a prone position (Fig. 8.2). The patient needs to turn prone to rise, then use their hands to climb up on their knees. Once at knee level, the hands are released, and the arms and body are swung sideways and upward to reach an upright position. Gower's sign is the typical symptom of Duchenne muscular dystrophy.

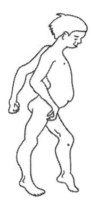

Figure 8.2. The symptoms of Duchenne muscular dystrophy.

There is currently no cure for DMD, but there are treatments that can help manage the symptoms and slow the progression of the disease. These may include medications, physical therapy, and assistive devices such as braces or wheelchairs.

Research is ongoing to develop new treatments for DMD, including gene therapy and other approaches to restore or replace dystrophin in muscle fibers. It is important for individuals with DMD to receive regular medical care and monitoring to manage the disease and optimize quality of life.

Myotonic dystrophy

Myotonic dystrophy is a genetic disorder that affects both the muscles and other body systems, including the heart, eyes, and brain. It is characterized by progressive muscle weakness and wasting, as well as myotonia, which is a delayed relaxation of the muscles after contraction. Myotonic dystrophy is caused by mutations in one of two genes, DMPK or CNBP.

There are two main types of myotonic dystrophy:

1. Myotonic dystrophy type 1 (DM1): This is the most common form of myotonic dystrophy, accounting for about 90% of cases. It is caused by mutations in the DMPK gene and is inherited in an autosomal dominant pattern. Symptoms of DM1 can vary widely, but typically include muscle weakness and wasting, myotonia, and other neurological and cognitive problems. Other symptoms may include cataracts, cardiac abnormalities, gastrointestinal problems, and endocrine disturbances.
2. Myotonic dystrophy type 2 (DM2): This is a less common form of myotonic dystrophy, accounting for about 10% of cases. It is caused by mutations in the CNBP gene and is also inherited in an autosomal dominant pattern. Symptoms of DM2 are similar to those of DM1, including muscle weakness and wasting, myotonia, and other neurological and cognitive problems. However, DM2 tends to be milder and progress more slowly than DM1.

There is currently no cure for myotonic dystrophy, but treatment can help manage the symptoms and improve quality of life.

Metabolic Myopathy

Metabolic myopathy is a type of skeletal muscle disease that results from a disruption in energy metabolism in muscle cells. It can be caused by inherited genetic mutations or acquired factors, and can affect individuals of any age.

1. Inherited forms of metabolic myopathy include glycogen storage disorders and lipid disorders. Glycogen storage disorders are caused by mutations in genes that encode enzymes involved in the breakdown and use of glycogen, a stored form of glucose that is used by muscles as a source of energy during exercise. Without sufficient glycogen breakdown, muscle cells cannot generate enough energy for muscle contractions, resulting in muscle weakness and fatigue. Lipid disorders involve defects in the metabolism of fats, which can lead to muscle damage and weakness.
2. Acquired forms of metabolic myopathy can result from a variety of factors, including exposure to toxins or drugs, vitamin deficiencies, or certain medical conditions such as diabetes or thyroid disease. These factors can interfere with the normal energy metabolism in muscle cells, leading to muscle weakness and other symptoms.

The symptoms of metabolic myopathy can vary widely depending on the specific underlying metabolic abnormality, but common features include muscle weakness, cramping, and fatigue.

Symptoms may be exacerbated by exercise or fasting, which increase the energy demands on muscle cells.

Diagnosis of metabolic myopathy typically involves a combination of clinical evaluation, laboratory testing, and genetic testing. Treatment options may include lifestyle modifications to avoid exacerbating factors, such as avoidance of fasting or certain medications, as well as medications to help manage symptoms and improve muscle function.

Polymyositis

Polymyositis is an inflammatory muscle disease that causes muscle weakness, particularly in the proximal muscles (muscles closest to the trunk of the body). It is a type of inflammatory myopathy and is believed to be an autoimmune disorder, meaning that the body's immune system mistakenly attacks and damages its own muscles.

The exact cause of polymyositis is unknown, but it is thought to be related to a combination of genetic and environmental factors. It can affect people of any age, but it most commonly occurs in adults between the ages of 40 and 60, and it affects women more frequently than men.

The main symptoms of polymyositis include progressive muscle weakness in the shoulders, hips, neck, and back, difficulty swallowing, and fatigue. Other symptoms can include muscle pain, tenderness, and stiffness. The severity of symptoms can vary from person to person and can range from mild to severe.

The diagnosis of polymyositis typically involves a thorough medical history, physical examination, and various tests, such as blood tests, electromyography (EMG), and muscle biopsy. Treatment typically involves the use of corticosteroids and other immunosuppressive medications to reduce inflammation and suppress the immune system's attack on the muscles. Physical therapy may also be helpful in improving muscle strength and function.

Early diagnosis and treatment of polymyositis are important for preventing long-term muscle damage and improving quality of life.

Alcohol-Induced Myopathy

An alcohol-induced myopathy is caused by excessive consumption of alcohol, which induces muscle toxicity.

There are two types of alcohol-induced myopathies:

1. *Acute alcohol-induced myopathy:* Acute alcohol-induced myopathy is due to a large amount of alcohol consumption in a short period. The symptoms include weakness, pain, tenderness, and swelling of affected muscles. Furthermore, the patient could have a substantial amount of myoglobulin passing through their urine. This is called *myoglobinuria*. In most cases, acute alcohol-induced myopathy is reversible.

2. *Sub-acute alcohol-induced proximal myopathy:* Sub-acute alcohol-induced proximal myopathy is due to the long-term consumption of an excessive amount of alcohol by patients. Myopathy is primarily in the proximal muscles, or *proximal myopathy*. Microscopic examination shows the histopathology of selective Type II muscle atrophy. Sub-acute alcohol-induced proximal myopathy is reversible in the early stage of the disease if alcohol consumption is limited.

Viral Myalgia

Viral myalgia is muscle pain or weakness caused by a viral infection. It is a common symptom of many viral illnesses, including the flu, COVID-19, and other respiratory infections. The muscle pain can be widespread or localized to specific areas of the body, and it can be severe enough to interfere with daily activities. In addition to muscle pain, viral myalgia may also cause other symptoms such as fever, fatigue, and headache. The muscle pain typically resolves on its own as the viral infection clears, but pain relief medications and rest may be helpful in managing symptoms.

Endocrine Myopathy

Endocrine myopathy is a type of myopathy that occurs due to an abnormality in the endocrine system, which is responsible for the secretion of hormones in the body. Hormones play a critical role in regulating many bodily functions, including muscle growth, maintenance, and repair. Therefore, when the endocrine system malfunctions and produces either too much or too little of certain hormones, it can lead to muscle weakness, fatigue, and wasting.

Examples of endocrine myopathies include:

1. Hypothyroid Myopathy: This occurs due to an underactive thyroid gland that results in decreased production of thyroid hormones. The muscle symptoms associated with hypothyroid myopathy include muscle weakness, cramping, stiffness, and slow movements.
2. Hyperthyroid Myopathy: This occurs due to an overactive thyroid gland that produces too much thyroid hormone. Muscle symptoms associated with hyperthyroid myopathy include muscle weakness, fatigue, and muscle wasting.
3. Cushing's Syndrome Myopathy: Cushing's syndrome is a condition that occurs due to an excess of cortisol, a hormone produced by the adrenal gland. The muscle symptoms associated with Cushing's syndrome myopathy include muscle weakness, fatigue, and muscle wasting.
4. Hyperparathyroidism Myopathy: This occurs due to an overactive parathyroid gland that produces too much parathyroid hormone. The muscle symptoms associated with hyperparathyroidism myopathy include muscle weakness, fatigue, and muscle wasting.

Muscle Tone Alteration

Muscle tonerefers to the natural resistance in muscles to passive movement. Alterations in muscle tone can occur in various neuromuscular and musculoskeletal disorders, resulting in changes in muscle stiffness or flaccidity.

1. Hypertonia: Hypertonia is an increase in muscle tone resulting in increased resistance to passive movement. This can be caused by upper motor neuron lesions, such as in cerebral palsy, stroke, or multiple sclerosis.
2. Hypotonia: Hypotonia is a decrease in muscle tone resulting in decreased resistance to passive movement. This can be caused by lower motor neuron lesions, such as in spinal muscular atrophy or myasthenia gravis, or in disorders affecting muscle, such as muscular dystrophies.
3. Rigidity: Rigidity is an increase in muscle tone that is uniform throughout the range of motion, and resistance to passive movement is felt in both directions. It can be caused by disorders affecting the basal ganglia, such as in Parkinson's disease.
4. Spasticity: Spasticity is a type of hypertonia that is characterized by increased resistance to passive movement, which is velocity-dependent, meaning that the resistance increases with increasing velocity of movement. It is caused by upper motor neuron lesions, such as in cerebral palsy, stroke, or multiple sclerosis.

5. Flaccidity: Flaccidity is a type of hypotonia that is characterized by a lack of muscle tone, resulting in a "floppy" appearance of the limbs. It can be caused by lower motor neuron lesions, such as in spinal muscular atrophy or myasthenia gravis, or in disorders affecting muscle, such as muscular dystrophies.

MUSCLE EXAMINATIONS

How to directly test muscle power?

Directly testing muscle power involves measuring the maximum amount of force that a muscle or muscle group can generate. Here are some methods to directly test muscle power:

1. Handheld dynamometry: This involves using a handheld device, such as a dynamometer, to measure the force produced by a muscle or muscle group. The patient is asked to push or pull against the device, and the force generated is measured in pounds or kilograms.

2. Isokinetic testing: This involves using a machine that controls the speed of joint movement to measure muscle strength throughout a range of motion. Isokinetic testing can measure peak torque, which is the maximum force generated by a muscle during a specific movement.

3. One-repetition maximum (1RM) testing: This involves determining the maximum amount of weight that a patient can

lift or move one time. This is commonly used in weightlifting and resistance training.

4. Functional testing: This involves testing the patient's ability to perform functional activities that require muscle power, such as jumping or running. The distance, speed, or time taken to complete the task can be used as a measure of muscle power.

It is important to note that directly testing muscle power requires specialized equipment and training, and should only be performed by qualified healthcare professionals.

Testing of voluntary muscle power

Direct testing of voluntary muscle power can be performed by asking the patient to push or pull in a specific direction against the examiner's resistance. The Medical Research Council (MRC) scale is commonly used to grade muscle strength based on the amount of resistance the patient can overcome during testing. The MRC scale ranges from 0 to 5, with 0 indicating no detectable muscle contraction and 5 indicating normal strength.

0: No movement or contraction is detected.
1. Muscle contraction is detected, but no movement occurs.
2. Movement occurs, but the patient is unable to overcome gravity.
3. The patient is able to move against gravity, but cannot overcome resistance.

4. The patient is able to move against gravity and overcome some resistance, but not full resistance.
5. The patient is able to move against gravity and overcome full resistance.

Indirect Testing of Muscle Power

Indirect testing of muscle power involves evaluating the functional abilities of the patient that are dependent on the strength of the muscles being tested. Indirect testing does not measure the strength of specific muscles or muscle groups directly, but instead assesses the patient's ability to perform activities that require the use of those muscles. Indirect testing can be used as a supplement to direct testing to provide a more comprehensive evaluation of muscle power.

Examples of indirect testing of muscle power include:

1. Timed up and go test: This test measures the time taken by a patient to stand up from a chair, walk a short distance, turn around, walk back to the chair and sit down again. It assesses the strength and balance of the lower limb muscles.
2. 6-minute walk test: This test measures the distance a patient can walk in 6 minutes. It assesses the strength and endurance of the lower limb muscles.
3. Hand grip strength test: This test measures the force a patient can generate with their hand grip using a hand-held

dynamometer. It assesses the strength of the hand and forearm muscles.

4. Functional Independence Measure (FIM): This is a standardized assessment tool that measures a patient's ability to perform activities of daily living, such as dressing, grooming, bathing, and toileting. It assesses the strength and functional abilities of various muscle groups throughout the body.

Indirect testing of muscle power can provide valuable information about a patient's overall muscle function and can be useful in identifying areas of weakness that may not be apparent from direct testing alone. It can also be used to monitor changes in muscle strength over time and to evaluate the effectiveness of rehabilitation programs.

Functional Testing of Muscle Power

Functional testing of muscle power involves evaluating the ability of the patient to perform specific functional tasks that require the use of multiple muscle groups. The aim of functional testing is to assess the patient's ability to perform activities of daily living and to identify any deficits that may be present.

Examples of functional testing of muscle power include:

1. Sit-to-stand test: This test measures the patient's ability to rise from a seated position without the use of their arms. It assesses the strength and endurance of the lower limb muscles.

2. Stair climb test: This test measures the patient's ability to ascend and descend a flight of stairs. It assesses the strength and endurance of the lower limb muscles and the patient's balance and coordination.

3. Carrying and lifting test: This test measures the patient's ability to carry and lift objects of varying weights and sizes. It assesses the strength and endurance of the upper limb and trunk muscles.

4. Balance and stability tests: These tests assess the patient's ability to maintain balance and stability in various positions, such as standing on one leg, walking on uneven surfaces, and turning around.

Functional testing of muscle power is important for assessing the patient's ability to perform activities of daily living and for identifying any areas of weakness or deficits in muscle function. It can also be used to monitor changes in muscle strength and functional abilities over time and to evaluate the effectiveness of rehabilitation programs.

Functional test and indirect test of muscle power

Functional testing of muscle power and indirect testing of muscle power are similar in that they both evaluate the patient's ability to perform activities that require the use of multiple muscle groups.

However, there are some differences between the two types of testing.

Indirect testing of muscle power typically involves the measurement of *a specific muscle or muscle group,* such as the hand grip strength test or the timed up and go test. The aim of indirect testing is to assess the strength of individual muscles or muscle groups and to identify any areas of weakness that may be present.

Functional testing of muscle power, on the other hand, involves evaluating the patient's ability to perform *functional tasks* that require the use of multiple muscle groups. The aim of functional testing is to assess the patient's ability to perform activities of daily living and to identify any deficits that may be present in their overall muscle function.

While there is some overlap between the two types of testing, functional testing of muscle power is typically more comprehensive than indirect testing and can provide a more complete evaluation of the patient's muscle function and functional abilities. Both types of testing can be useful in assessing the patient's muscle power and in developing an appropriate rehabilitation plan.

Examinations of the muscle shape and size

Examination of the shape and size of muscles can provide valuable information about the patient's muscle function and any underlying conditions that may be present. There are several methods that can be used to examine the shape and size of muscles, including:

1. Inspection: Visual inspection of the patient's muscles can provide information about their shape and size. For example, atrophy or wasting of the muscles may be evident in certain conditions such as muscular dystrophy or peripheral neuropathy.

2. Palpation: Palpation involves feeling the patient's muscles with the hands to assess their size, texture, and tone. The examiner can also check for any areas of tenderness, swelling, or deformity.

3. Circumference measurements: Measurements of the circumference of specific muscle groups can provide information about their size and any changes that may have occurred. For example, a decrease in the circumference of the calf muscles may indicate muscle wasting.

4. Imaging studies: Imaging studies such as magnetic resonance imaging (MRI) or ultrasound can provide detailed information about the shape and size of muscles and any underlying abnormalities or pathology.

Examination of the shape and size of muscles can be useful in identifying areas of weakness or atrophy and in determining the underlying cause of muscle dysfunction. It can also be used to monitor changes in muscle size and function over time and to evaluate the effectiveness of rehabilitation programs.

Fasciculation

Fasciculations are involuntary muscle contractions that can be seen or felt as small twitching movements under the skin. Examination of fasciculations can provide important diagnostic information about the patient's neuromuscular function. Here are the steps to examine fasciculations:

1. Visual inspection: The examiner should observe the affected muscles for any visible twitching or movement. This can be done in a well-lit room with the patient at rest or during muscle activation.
2. Palpation: The examiner should feel the affected muscles for any areas of twitching or movement. This can be done with the fingers or by using a stethoscope to listen for muscle activity.
3. Provocative maneuvers: The examiner may perform certain maneuvers to provoke or enhance fasciculations. For example, tapping or percussing the affected muscle may induce fasciculations.
4. Electromyography (EMG): EMG is a diagnostic test that can be used to evaluate muscle and nerve function. It involves placing small electrodes into the muscle to record electrical activity. EMG can be used to confirm the presence of fasciculations and to determine their underlying cause.

Examination of fasciculations can provide important diagnostic information about the patient's neuromuscular function. It can be used to diagnose conditions such as amyotrophic lateral sclerosis (ALS), peripheral neuropathy, or other neuromuscular disorders. If fasciculations are observed, further evaluation may be necessary to determine the underlying cause and develop an appropriate treatment plan.

Muscle Tone

Muscle tone is the resistance of a muscle to passive movement. Examination of muscle tone involves assessing the degree of resistance to passive movement in a relaxed muscle. Here are the steps to examine muscle tone:

1. Positioning: The patient should be positioned in a comfortable and relaxed position. The muscle group being tested should be exposed and the patient should be instructed to relax.

2. Palpation: The examiner should palpate the muscle group being tested to assess its overall tone and any areas of hypertonicity or spasticity.

3. Passive range of motion: The examiner should move the patient's joint through a full range of motion to assess the degree of resistance to passive movement. The examiner should note any areas of increased or decreased resistance.

4. Modified Ashworth Scale: The Modified Ashworth Scale is a commonly used tool to assess muscle tone. The examiner rates the degree of resistance to passive movement on a scale from 0-4, with 0 indicating no resistance and 4 indicating rigidity.

5. Other testing methods: Other testing methods, such as the pendulum test or the stretch reflex test, may be used to assess muscle tone in specific muscle groups.

Examination of muscle tone can provide important diagnostic information about the patient's neuromuscular function. It can be used to diagnose conditions such as cerebral palsy, stroke, or other neurological disorders. Treatment for abnormal muscle tone may include physical therapy, medication, or surgery.

Cogwheel rigidity

Cogwheel rigidity is a neurological symptom that can occur in Parkinson's disease and some other movement disorders. It refers to the stiffness or resistance of movement that is felt when trying to move a limb or joint.

Cogwheel rigidity is caused by an abnormality in the basal ganglia. Specifically, it is thought to result from an imbalance between the neurotransmitters dopamine and acetylcholine, which are both involved in regulating movement.

The term "cogwheel" refers to the sensation of movement being obstructed or interrupted, as if the joint were moving in a series of small steps, like the teeth of a cogwheel. This type of rigidity is usually most prominent in the arms, but can also occur in the legs or other parts of the body.

Cogwheel rigidity can be assessed by a neurologist during a physical examination, and is often treated with medications that help to restore the balance of dopamine and acetylcholine in the brain.

CHAPTER 9: UPPER LIMB MOTOR DYSFUNCTION

Upper limb motor dysfunction refers to a broad range of motor impairments that can affect the arms, hands, and fingers. These impairments can result from a variety of neurological or musculoskeletal conditions, including stroke, spinal cord injury, multiple sclerosis, cerebral palsy, and Parkinson's disease.

Some common signs of upper limb motor dysfunction include weakness, spasticity (muscle stiffness and involuntary contractions), tremors, decreased range of motion, and difficulty with coordination and fine motor tasks. These impairments can significantly impact an individual's ability to perform activities of daily living, such as dressing, grooming, and eating.

Treatment options for upper limb motor dysfunction depend on the underlying condition and the severity of the impairment. Physical therapy and occupational therapy are often recommended to improve range of motion, strength, and coordination. Other interventions may include medication to reduce spasticity or tremors, assistive devices to aid with mobility and daily activities, and surgery in some cases.

NERVE INJURY

Peripheral nerve injury refers to damage to the nerves outside of the brain and spinal cord, which can result in a wide range of symptoms depending on the location and severity of the injury. Peripheral nerves are responsible for carrying messages between the brain and the rest of the body, including sensations such as touch and pain, as well as motor signals that control muscle movements.

Peripheral nerve injuries can be caused by a variety of factors, including trauma, infection, exposure to toxins, and certain medical conditions. Common examples of peripheral nerve injuries include carpal tunnel syndrome, which is caused by compression of the median nerve in the wrist, and sciatica, which is caused by compression of the sciatic nerve in the lower back.

Symptoms of peripheral nerve injury can include numbness, tingling, weakness, pain, and muscle atrophy (wasting). The severity of these symptoms can vary depending on the extent of the nerve damage and the location of the injury.

Treatment for peripheral nerve injury depends on the severity of the injury and the underlying cause. In some cases, rest and immobilization may be sufficient to allow the nerve to heal on its own. In other cases, surgery or other medical interventions may be necessary to repair or replace damaged nerve tissue. Physical therapy may also be recommended to help improve strength, range of motion, and overall function.

Spinal nerves and motor dysfunction

Spinal nerves are the nerves that originate from the spinal cord and transmit sensory and motor information between the body and the central nervous system. There are 31 pairs of spinal nerves that exit the spinal cord and are named according to the level of the vertebrae they originate from.

Motor dysfunction can occur when there is damage or injury to the spinal nerves, which can lead to weakness, paralysis, or muscle atrophy in the affected area. The specific symptoms and severity of motor dysfunction depend on the location and extent of the nerve damage.

For example, damage to the spinal nerves in the cervical (neck) region can cause motor dysfunction in the arms and hands, while damage to the spinal nerves in the lumbar (lower back) region can cause motor dysfunction in the legs and feet.

Common causes of spinal nerve damage include trauma, herniated discs, spinal stenosis (narrowing of the spinal canal), and degenerative disc disease. Certain medical conditions such as multiple sclerosis, spinal cord tumors, and Guillain-Barre syndrome can also affect the spinal nerves and cause motor dysfunction.

Cranial Nerves and motor dysfunction

The cranial nerves are a set of 12 pairs of nerves that originate in the brain and innervate various structures in the head, neck, and upper torso. Each cranial nerve is responsible for specific functions related to sensation, motor control, or both.

Motor dysfunction related to cranial nerves can result from damage or dysfunction of one or more cranial nerves. This can lead to a variety of symptoms depending on which nerve is affected. Some examples include:

- Cranial nerve III (oculomotor nerve): Damage to this nerve can cause weakness or paralysis of eye muscles, leading to symptoms such as double vision or drooping eyelids.
- Cranial nerve VII (facial nerve): Damage to this nerve can result in facial weakness or paralysis, causing difficulty with facial expressions, drooping of the eyelid or mouth, or difficulty with speech and swallowing.
- Cranial nerve X (vagus nerve): Damage to this nerve can cause difficulty with swallowing or speaking, hoarseness, or weakness of the palate, resulting in difficulty with swallowing or speaking.

Treatment for motor dysfunction related to cranial nerves depends on the underlying cause and severity of the injury. In some cases, rest and rehabilitation may be sufficient to restore function. In other cases, medical interventions such as medication, surgery, or physical therapy may be necessary.

Brachial Plexus Injuries

A brachial plexus injury is a type of nerve injury that affects the nerves that control movement and sensation in the shoulder, arm, and hand. The brachial plexus is a network of nerves that originates from the spinal cord in the neck and extends into the upper extremity.

Brachial plexus injuries can occur as a result of trauma, such as during a motor vehicle accident, sports injury, or a fall (Fig. 9.1). They can also occur during childbirth, particularly if there is difficulty delivering the baby's shoulder.

The symptoms of brachial plexus injury vary depending on the severity of the injury. Mild injuries may cause temporary weakness or numbness in the affected area, while more severe injuries can cause permanent paralysis or loss of sensation.

Motor dysfunction is a common symptom of brachial plexus injury and can manifest as weakness, paralysis, or muscle atrophy in the affected arm or hand. The specific symptoms depend on the location and extent of the nerve damage.

Chapter 9: Upper Limb Motor Dysfunction

Treatment for brachial plexus injury depends on the severity of the injury and the specific symptoms. Mild injuries may not require treatment and may resolve on their own over time. In more severe cases, surgery may be necessary to repair or reconstruct damaged nerves.

Physical therapy and occupational therapy can also be helpful in improving strength, mobility, and overall function. Assistive devices such as braces or splints may be recommended to help with support and mobility.

Injuries to the supraclavicular part of the brachial plexus

Injury to the supraclavicular part of the brachial plexus can cause significant motor dysfunction in the shoulder, arm, and hand. It occurs as a result of excessive stretching or compression of the nerves that control these areas. This can happen due to a variety of causes, including falls from a high position or trauma to the neck and shoulder region.

In newborns, injuries to the supraclavicular part of the brachial plexus can occur during delivery if the baby's head is pulled in a lateral direction.

Symptoms of injuries to the supraclavicular part of the brachial plexus include an adducted shoulder and an extended elbow, which causes the patient to exhibit a "Waiter's tip position" with the limb hanging by the side in a medial rotation position of the arm. This position indicates weakness in the deltoid, biceps, brachialis, and brachioradialis muscles. Sensation is lost in the lateral aspect of the upper limbs, primarily affecting the skin region supplied by the C5 and C6 levels of the spinal cord.

Treatment for injuries to the supraclavicular part of the brachial plexus depends on the severity of the injury and the specific symptoms. Mild injuries may require rest and physical therapy, while more severe injuries may require surgery to repair or reconstruct damaged nerves. Physical therapy and occupational therapy can also be helpful in improving strength, mobility, and overall function. Assistive devices such as braces or splints may be recommended to help with support and mobility.

Early diagnosis and treatment are important in maximizing the chances of recovery from injuries to the supraclavicular part of the brachial plexus and reducing the risk of long-term motor dysfunction. If you experience symptoms of motor dysfunction following an injury to the supraclavicular part of the brachial plexus, it is essential to seek medical attention promptly to determine the underlying cause and appropriate treatment options.

Chapter 9: Upper Limb Motor Dysfunction

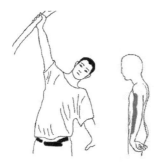

Figure 9.1. Brachial plexus injury.

Injuries to the Infraclavicular Part of the Brachial Plexus

Injuries to the infraclavicular part of the brachial plexus can occur when the upper limb is suddenly pulled upward, as may happen when a person grabs a tree branch during a fall. This sudden upward pull can cause damage to the brachial plexus. Additionally, during birth, the infant's arm may be excessively pulled, resulting in injury to the inferior part of the brachial plexus.

Symptoms of injuries to the infraclavicular part of the brachial plexus are primarily related to the C7, C8, and T1 levels of the spinal cord. The muscles in the hand, including the short muscles, are often affected, resulting in a "claw-hand" appearance. In this condition, the fingers are hyperextended at the metacarpophalangeal joints and flexed at the interphalangeal joints, giving the hand a claw-like appearance.

In addition to motor dysfunction, injuries to the infraclavicular part of the brachial plexus may also cause sensory changes, such as loss of sensation or abnormal sensations in the affected limb. Pain, weakness, and difficulty with movement may also be present.

Treatment for injuries to the infraclavicular part of the brachial plexus may include physical therapy, occupational therapy, and/or surgical intervention, depending on the severity of the injury and the specific symptoms. Physical therapy and occupational therapy can help improve strength, mobility, and overall function. Surgical intervention may be required to repair or reconstruct damaged nerves.

Hyperabduction syndrome

Hyperabduction syndrome is a condition that occurs when the brachial plexus, a network of nerves that controls movement and sensation in the arm, is compressed during activities that involve lifting the arm above the head. For example, while painting a ceiling, the cord of the brachial plexus can be compressed between the coracoid process of the scapula and the tendon of the pectoralis minor.

Compression of the brachial plexus can also cause compression of the axillary artery and veins, which can lead to a lack of blood supply to the upper limbs and distension of the veins. The resulting symptoms of hyperabduction syndrome include pain running down the arm, numbness, tingling, and weakness in the hands.

Additionally, the skin in the affected area may become red due to capillary dilation.

Diagnosis of hyperabduction syndrome typically involves a physical examination and imaging tests such as X-rays, CT scans, or MRI scans. Treatment options may include physical therapy, medications for pain and inflammation, and in severe cases, surgery to relieve the compression of the brachial plexus.

Prevention of hyperabduction syndrome involves proper body mechanics and technique during activities that involve lifting the arm above the head, as well as taking frequent breaks and stretching to prevent overuse and fatigue of the muscles in the shoulder and arm.

Axillary Nerve Injury

Axillary nerve injury is characterized by paralysis of the deltoid muscle and can be caused by a variety of factors. The axillary nerve is derived from the C5 and C6 levels of the spinal cord and supplies the deltoid and teres minor muscles, as well as the skin over the inferior part of the deltoid muscle and shoulder joint.

The most common causes of axillary nerve injury include bone fracture of the neck of the humerus, as the axillary nerve passes posteriorly around the surgical neck of the humerus, and joint dislocation of the shoulder joint. Injections of drugs into the deltoid muscle can also injure the axillary nerve, particularly if the injection is administered too deeply, as the axillary nerve supplying the deltoid muscle runs transversely under the cover of the deltoid muscle.

Symptoms of axillary nerve injury include paralysis and atrophy of the deltoid muscle, which can result in a flattened appearance of the shoulder joint inferior to the acromion. The patient may also experience a loss of sensation over the lateral side of the proximal part of the arm, as this area is supplied by the sensory component of the axillary nerve. Additionally, the patient may have difficulty performing arm abductions due to the lack of axillary nerves supplying the deltoid and teres minor muscles.

Long Thoracic Nerve Injury

The long thoracic nerve originates from the spinal cord segments C5, C6, and C7 and is responsible for supplying the serratus anterior muscle. The nerve runs between the superficial layer of the serratus anterior muscle and the skin, making it vulnerable to injury.

Causes of Long Thoracic Nerve Injury: The most common cause of long thoracic nerve injury is trauma, such as a knife or gunshot wound. The nerve is particularly susceptible to damage when the arm is elevated and left unprotected.

Symptoms of Long Thoracic Nerve Injury: The primary symptom of long thoracic nerve injury is winged scapula, which occurs when the serratus anterior muscle is paralyzed due to nerve damage. As a result, the medial border of the scapula moves laterally and posteriorly, giving the scapula a wing-like appearance. This symptom is more pronounced when the person leans on an elbow or places a hand against a wall. Additionally, the patient may experience difficulty in raising their arm above the horizontal position.

Median Nerve Injury

The median nerve originates from the spinal cord's C6, C7, C8, and T1 segments. It runs laterally to the axillary artery and passes anteriorly to the inferior part of the humerus in the cubital fossa. The median nerve innervates the flexor muscles of the forearm (excluding flexor carpi ulnaris and the ulnar half of the flexor digitorum profundus) and five hand muscles.

Median nerve injury can occur at either the elbow or wrist region, with the most common site being the carpal tunnel.

Symptoms of Median Nerve Injury can include:

1. Abnormality of the distal interphalangeal joint: Patients lose flexion of the distal interphalangeal (DIP) joints of the second and third digits. However, flexion of the DIP joints of the fourth and fifth digits is not affected because the medial part of the flexor digitorum profundus (DFP) is supplied by the ulnar nerve.

2. Abnormality of the proximal interphalangeal joint: Patients lose flexion of the proximal interphalangeal (PIP) joints of digits one to three. The flexion of digits four and five is weakened.

3. Abnormality of the metacarpophalangeal joint: The distal branches of the median nerve supply the first and second lumbricals, which affects the flexion of the metacarpophalangeal joints of the second and third digits.

4. Hand of Benediction: Median nerve injury can also lead to weakness of the thenar muscles, resulting in a hand of benediction appearance (Fig. 9.2).

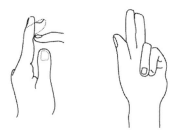

Figure 9.2. Hand of benediction. The figure shows the testing flexion of the flexor muscles of the digits (on the left). The hand of benediction (on the right) is a sign of median nerve injury.

Radial Nerve Injury

The radial nerve originates from the spinal cord's C5 to C8 and T1 segments and passes through the radial groove, located between the long and medial heads of the triceps. It supplies the triceps brachii, anconeus, brachioradialis, and extensor muscles in the forearm, as well as the skin on the posterior aspect of the arm and forearm via the posterior cutaneous nerve.

Causes of Radial Nerve Injury: The most common cause of radial nerve injury is a humeral shaft fracture.

Symptoms of Radial Nerve Injury: Wrist Drop and Flexed Digits: Typically, the injury occurs proximal to the branches of the forearm muscles and wrist extensors, resulting in wrist drop as the primary clinical manifestation of radial nerve injury (Fig. 9.3). The patient will be unable to extend the wrist and digits, and the muscles in the posterior compartment of the forearm, supplied by distal branches of the nerve, will be paralyzed. The triceps will be weakened as a result of medial head involvement. The patient may experience minimal loss of sensation distal to the base of the first and second metacarpals.

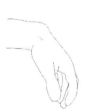

Figure 9.3. Wrist-drop sign as seen in radial nerve injury. The patient cannot extend the wrist as the muscles in the posterior compartment of the forearm are paralyzed because of the radial nerve injury.

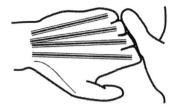

Figure 9.4. Test of the function of the extensor muscles of the digits. The patient with a radial nerve injury cannot extend the digits. If it is a minor injury, muscle weakness can be seen.

Ulnar Nerve Injury

The ulnar nerve originates from the C8 and T1 segments of the spinal cord. It courses down the arm's medial aspect, passing posterior to the medial epicondyle, and enters the forearm. The ulnar nerve supplies the flexor carpi ulnaris, the medial half of the flexor digitorum profundus, and the intrinsic muscles of the hand, as well as the skin of the hand medial to the fourth digit (Fig. 73).

CAUSES: Ulnar nerve injury is commonly caused by trauma to the medial part of the elbow, such as a fracture of the medial epicondyle (funny bone), olecranon, or head of the radius. It can also result from gunshot and stab wounds. Ulnar nerve injuries constitute about 30% of nerve lesions of the upper limbs.

SYMPTOMS: Sensory abnormalities: Patients experience numbness and tingling in the medial part of the palm and the medial one-and-a-half digits. They may also have elbow pain that radiates distally.

Chapter 9: Upper Limb Motor Dysfunction

Motor abnormalities: Ulnar nerve injury affects the intrinsic muscles of the hand, resulting in weakness and atrophy of the hypothenar muscles, the interossei, and the medial two lumbricals. The patient may have difficulty making a fist because they cannot flex the fourth and fifth digits at the distal interphalangeal joints. Additionally, the patient's grip strength is weakened, and the power of adduction of the hand is impaired.

Hand appearance: Claw hand is a characteristic feature of patients after ulnar nerve injury (Fig. 9.6). The fourth and fifth digits are extended at the metacarpophalangeal joints and flexed at the proximal and distal interphalangeal joints. Patients cannot extend their interphalangeal joints when they try to straighten their fingers. Furthermore, the metacarpophalangeal joints become overextended, making it difficult for the patient to grip objects because of the paralysis of most of the intrinsic hand muscles.

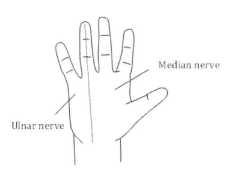

Figure 9.5. Area of a hand and fingers supplied by the ulnar nerve. The figure shows the area of a hand and fingers supplied

by the ulnar nerve. Ulnar nerve injury causes a loss of superficial sensation in the area left of the dotted line.

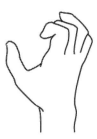

Figure 9.6. The appearance of a claw hand, which can be seen after an ulnar nerve injury.

Chapter 9: Upper Limb Motor Dysfunction

JOINT INJURY

Upper limb joint injuries can lead to motor dysfunction, which refers to a loss or impairment of movement or coordination. Depending on the specific joint affected and the severity of the injury, different types of motor dysfunction can occur.

For example, a rotator cuff tear or shoulder dislocation can result in weakness and limited range of motion in the shoulder joint, making it difficult to lift or move the arm. A wrist sprain can cause difficulty with fine motor movements, such as grasping and holding objects. An elbow dislocation or tennis elbow can lead to pain and weakness in the arm and difficulty with gripping and lifting.

In some cases, motor dysfunction resulting from an upper limb joint injury may be temporary and improve with rest, physical therapy, and other forms of rehabilitation. However, in more severe cases, surgery may be necessary to repair the joint and restore function.

Overall, the best course of treatment for upper limb joint injuries and resulting motor dysfunction will depend on the specific type and severity of the injury, as well as the individual's overall health and medical history. It is important to work closely with a healthcare professional to develop an appropriate treatment plan and to follow through with recommended rehabilitation and therapy to promote healing and improve function.

Joint

A joint is an articulation between the bones. The degree of movement varies according to how the articulation is formed. Some joints, such as fibrous and cartilaginous joints, allow slight or no movement. Others are freely movable, such as synovial joints.

Joint injury is a common cause of motor dysfunction and is mainly due to the dislocation of the articular surfaces, called *joint dislocation*. The main symptoms of joint dislocation are movement restriction and pain caused by hemorrhage of blood vessels and swelling of soft tissue injuries. Inflammation can also occur after a joint injury.

Fibrous, cartilaginous, and synovial joints

The human body contains three types of joints: fibrous, cartilaginous, and synovial.

Fibrous joints are connected by fibrous connective tissue and can be immovable or only allow limited movement. There are three types of fibrous joints:

1. Suture joints, which are tightly connected by dense connective tissues and can be found between the cranial bones.

2. Syndesmosis joints, which are connected by a ligament and membrane and are located between the tibia and fibula bones.

Chapter 9: Upper Limb Motor Dysfunction

3. Gomphosis joints, which occur where a cone-shaped end fits into a complementary socket held by a ligament. For example, teeth in their sockets form gomphosis joints.

Cartilaginous joints are connected by fibrous cartilage or hyaline cartilage. There are two types of cartilaginous joints:

1. Synchondrosis joints, which are connected by hyaline cartilage. Synchondrosis joints can be found between the rib and sternum.

2. Symphysis joints, which are connected by fibrous cartilage. Symphysis joints are found between the two pubic bones and the intervertebral disks.

The most common type of joint in the body is the synovial joint, which allows for a wide range of movement. Synovial joints are surrounded by a joint capsule and contain synovial fluid, which lubricates the joint and reduces friction. Examples of synovial joints include the shoulder, elbow, wrist, hip, knee, and ankle.

Understanding the anatomy of joints is essential for diagnosing and treating joint disorders and injuries. It can also help prevent injuries by promoting proper joint movement and stability during physical activities.

Structures of Synovial Joint

Synovial joints are complex structures that allow for a wide range of movement. The following are the key structures of synovial joints:

- Articular surfaces: These are the surfaces of the bones that come together to form the joint. All articular surfaces are covered by articular cartilage, which provides a smooth and slippery surface for joint movement.
- Articular capsule: This is a fibrous connective tissue that surrounds the joint, providing stability and protecting the joint from injury. The synovial membrane is a layer of soft connective tissue lining the inside of the capsule and secretes synovial fluid.
- Articular cavity and fluid: The articular cavity is a space inside the synovial capsule that is filled with synovial fluid. This fluid lubricates the joint, reduces friction between the articular surfaces, and provides nutrients and oxygen to the joint.
- Ligaments: These are dense connective tissues that connect bone to bone and enhance the stability of the joint. Ligaments are responsible for preventing excessive or abnormal movement of the joint.
- Articular disk: This is a cartilaginous plate that is found in some synovial joints, such as the knee joint. The disk provides additional stability and helps distribute weight evenly across the joint.

- Articular labrum: The labrum is a cartilage rim that surrounds the edge of the articular surface. It increases the depth of the articular surface, providing additional stability and reducing the risk of dislocation. The labrum is found in the shoulder and hip joints.

Understanding the structures of synovial joints is important for maintaining joint health and preventing joint injuries. It can also aid in the diagnosis and treatment of joint disorders and injuries.

Movements of the Joints

Joints are capable of a wide range of movements that can be categorized into three main types based on the number of axes involved:

1. Uniaxial movement: This type of joint can move in one plane or dimension only. Examples include the elbow joint, which allows for flexion and extension only along the sagittal plane.
2. Biaxial movement: This type of joint can move in two planes or dimensions. Examples include the finger joints, which allow for flexion and extension along the sagittal plane, as well as adduction and abduction along the coronal plane.
3. Multiaxial movement: This type of joint can move in all three planes or dimensions. Examples include the shoulder and hip joints, which allow for flexion and extension along the sagittal

plane, adduction and abduction along the coronal plane, and rotation along the transverse plane.

In addition to these categories, joints can also have a combination of movements, such as the wrist joint, which is capable of flexion, extension, adduction, abduction, and circumduction. Understanding the different types of joint movements is important for both functional activities and injury prevention.

Joint dislocation

Joint dislocation can be a significant cause of motor dysfunction, and it can occur at any age. However, clinically, joint dislocations are more common in individuals under the age of twenty.

There are several possible causes of joint dislocation, including:

- Trauma: Joint dislocations are often the result of traumatic events such as car accidents, sports injuries, or physical altercations.
- Congenital joint dislocation: This type of joint abnormality is hereditary and can be seen in hip joint dislocation. Patients with congenital joint dislocation often exhibit both muscle weakness and an abnormality in the shape of the articular surface.
- Neurological disorders: Joint function can be affected by both motor and sensory nerve injuries, making joints with neurological disorders more susceptible to dislocation.

- Pathological causes: Damage to the articulating surface, such as that seen in rheumatoid arthritis, can lead to joint dysfunction and an increased risk of dislocation.

Dislocation of a joint can cause significant motor dysfunction, including pain, weakness, and loss of range of motion. Treatment typically involves reducing the dislocation, managing pain and inflammation, and performing physical therapy to restore joint function. In some cases, surgery may be necessary to repair damaged tissues and stabilize the joint.

Clinical manifestations of joint injury

- Pain: Joint dislocation commonly causes pain, which can result from damage to soft tissues, arteries, veins, nerves, and muscles.
- Swelling: Hemorrhage and inflammation caused by joint dislocation can result in soft tissue swelling.
- Limited range of motion: Patients with joint dislocation may experience limited range of motion, which can also be due to pain.
- Joint deformity: Joint dislocation can alter the shape of the joint, causing the position of the articular surface to shift. This can be observed through altered bony landmarks in the joint. Muscle contraction around the joint can also cause changes in the joint's appearance after dislocation.

It is worth noting that clinical manifestations can vary depending on the severity of the joint injury and other contributing factors such as age, underlying health conditions, and type of joint affected.

General Pathology of Joint Dislocation

Joint dislocation can cause various pathological changes, including:

1. Soft tissue injuries: Dislocated joints often cause damage to nearby ligaments, tendons, nerves, and blood vessels. The extent of the injury depends on the severity of the dislocation.

2. Bone fracture: Joint dislocation can sometimes cause bone fractures near the joint. Fractures can be minor or severe and may require additional treatment.

3. Cartilage damage: Dislocated joints can also damage the articular cartilage that covers the bones' surfaces. Cartilage damage can lead to joint instability, pain, and arthritis in the future.

Treatment of Joint Dislocation

The immediate treatment for joint dislocation is the reduction of the dislocated joint, which involves moving the bone back into its normal position. After reduction, the joint is immobilized with a splint, cast, or sling for a period of two to six weeks. This immobilization allows the soft tissues and bone to heal and prevents the joint from moving and causing further damage. Physical therapy may also be recommended to help restore joint function and strength. In severe cases or when there is significant damage to the joint, surgery may be required.

General Pathology of Joint Dislocation

Joint dislocation can cause several pathologies, including:

- One displacement: the articular surface of the joint is moved from its normal position, which can damage the surrounding tissues.
- Injuries to nerves and ligaments adjacent to the dislocated joint: the displacement of the joint can cause stretching, tearing, or compression of the nerves and ligaments surrounding it, leading to pain and dysfunction.
- Bruising due to blood vessel damage: the displacement of the joint can damage blood vessels, causing internal bleeding and bruising.
- Bone fracture: joint dislocation can sometimes cause fractures in the adjacent bones, which can complicate the recovery process.
- Damage to the hyaline cartilage: the articular cartilage covering the bone ends of the joint can be damaged or even torn during a dislocation.

Shoulder joint dislocation

Shoulder joint dislocation is a condition that occurs when the upper arm bone (humerus) is forced out of the shoulder socket (glenoid). This usually happens due to a traumatic injury or a fall. Shoulder joint dislocation is more common in young adults, especially those involved in contact sports such as football or rugby.

The symptoms of a shoulder joint dislocation include severe pain, swelling, and deformity of the shoulder. The arm may also feel numb or tingly, and there may be difficulty moving the shoulder.

The treatment of shoulder joint dislocation involves reducing the dislocation, which means placing the humerus back into the glenoid socket. This is often done under sedation or anesthesia in a hospital setting. After the reduction, the shoulder will be immobilized with a sling or brace for several weeks to allow the ligaments and tissues to heal. Physical therapy is also recommended to restore shoulder strength and flexibility.

If shoulder joint dislocation occurs repeatedly, surgery may be necessary to repair or reconstruct the damaged ligaments and tissues in the shoulder joint.

Chapter 9: Upper Limb Motor Dysfunction

Anterior dislocation of the shoulder joint

Anterior dislocation of the shoulder joint, also known as a subcoracoid dislocation, is a common type of shoulder dislocation. It occurs when the humeral head (the ball-shaped end of the upper arm bone) is displaced in front of the glenoid (the shallow socket of the shoulder blade).

This can cause the humeral head to be forced out of the glenoid fossa and result in dislocation. Certain sports activities, such as football, hockey, and skiing, can also increase the risk of shoulder dislocation. In some cases, repetitive overhead movements or hypermobility of the joint can contribute to the development of shoulder instability, which can lead to dislocation. This can result from a sudden forceful movement or trauma to the shoulder, such as a fall, sports injury, or car accident.

The clinical manifestations of an anterior shoulder dislocation include severe pain, swelling, and limited range of motion. The arm may appear to be out of position, and the patient may have difficulty moving the shoulder or using the affected arm. Numbness or tingling in the arm or hand may also be present if nerves are affected.

Immediate treatment for an anterior shoulder dislocation involves reducing the dislocation by gently manipulating the humeral head back into its proper position. This is typically done under sedation or anesthesia to reduce pain and muscle spasms. After reduction, the shoulder is immobilized in a sling or brace for several weeks to allow for healing and prevent re-dislocation. Physical therapy may also be recommended to restore strength and range of motion to the affected shoulder.

Posterior dislocation of the shoulder joint

Posterior dislocation of the shoulder joint is less common than anterior dislocation and accounts for only about 2-4% of all shoulder dislocations. It occurs when the humeral head moves posteriorly (backwards) out of the glenoid fossa of the scapula. This type of dislocation is usually caused by a force applied to the anterior aspect of the shoulder while the arm is in a forward, elevated, and internally rotated position. This can occur in sports like football, rugby, and wrestling, as well as from falls or motor vehicle accidents. Other risk factors include a history of shoulder instability or laxity, repetitive overhead activities, and certain medical conditions such as epilepsy or cerebral palsy. Posterior dislocation of the shoulder joint can also be associated with fractures of the humerus or scapula.

Complications of shoulder joint dislocation

Complications of shoulder joint dislocation can vary depending on the severity of the injury and the duration of the dislocation. Some common complications include:

Chapter 9: Upper Limb Motor Dysfunction

1. Recurrent dislocation: Patients who have experienced shoulder joint dislocation are at risk for recurrent dislocation, especially if they have not received appropriate treatment or rehabilitation.

2. Rotator cuff injuries: The rotator cuff is a group of muscles and tendons that stabilize the shoulder joint. A dislocation can cause tears or strains in these structures, leading to pain and weakness in the shoulder.

3. Labral tears: The labrum is a ring of cartilage that surrounds the rim of the shoulder socket, providing stability to the joint. A dislocation can cause tears in the labrum, which can lead to recurrent instability.

4. Nerve damage: The nerves that supply sensation and motor function to the arm and hand can be stretched or compressed during a dislocation, leading to temporary or permanent weakness, numbness, or tingling.

5. Frozen shoulder: This is a condition where the shoulder becomes stiff and painful, limiting range of motion. It can occur after a dislocation due to inflammation and scarring around the joint.

6. Osteoarthritis: Over time, repeated dislocations or injuries to the shoulder joint can lead to degeneration of the cartilage and bone, resulting in osteoarthritis.

Acromioclavicular Joint dislocation

Anatomy of the Acromioclavicular Joint: The acromioclavicular joint is formed by the acromion process of the scapula and the lateral end of the clavicle bone. The joint is stabilized by three main ligaments: the coracoclavicular ligament, which is divided into two parts - the conoid part medially and the trapezoid part laterally; the acromioclavicular ligament, which reinforces the joint capsule superiorly; and the coracoacromial ligament, which is attached to the coracoid process of the scapula and the acromion process.

Causes: Acromioclavicular joint dislocation typically occurs due to direct trauma to the shoulder, such as a fall on an outstretched hand, a collision, or a blow to the top of the shoulder. It can also occur due to repetitive stress on the joint, as seen in sports that involve overhead motions such as throwing or weightlifting.

Pathology: Acromioclavicular joint dislocation refers to the separation of the acromion and clavicle bones that form the joint. Depending on the severity of the dislocation, the ligaments that support the joint may also be damaged or torn.

Symptoms: The most common symptom of acromioclavicular joint dislocation is pain in the shoulder region, particularly on the most lateral upper part of the shoulder. The dislocation may also result in an apparent prominence or bump in the area where the clavicle meets the acromion, and a dropped shoulder may be present. Additionally, patients may experience limited range of motion and weakness in the affected arm.

Chapter 9: Upper Limb Motor Dysfunction

Elbow Joint Dislocation

Anatomy: The elbow joint is composed of two articular surfaces, namely the humeroulnar joint formed by the trochlea of the humerus and the trochlear notch of the ulna, and the humeroradial joint formed by the humeral capitulum and the radial head. The ligaments of the elbow joint include the ulnar collateral (medial collateral) ligament, radial collateral ligament, and annular ligament.

Causes: Elbow joint dislocation, also known as "pulled elbow," is commonly observed in preschool children. It usually occurs due to a sudden arm lift, especially when the child has their forearm in a pronated position.

Symptoms: Elbow joint dislocation can cause the following symptoms:

- Displacement of the three bony landmarks, including the medial epicondyle, lateral epicondyle, and olecranon process. Normally, these three bony marks form a straight line when the elbow joint is extended. In a child with elbow dislocation, the olecranon process is located distal to the medial and lateral epicondyles of the humerus.

- The child's elbow may show the olecranon process located proximal to the medial and lateral epicondyles when the elbow joint is flexed.

Proper diagnosis and treatment are necessary for elbow joint dislocation. If you suspect an elbow dislocation, seek medical attention immediately.

BONE FRACTURE

Upper limb bone fractures can lead to motor dysfunction due to the disruption of the normal functioning of the bones, joints, and muscles involved in upper limb movement. These fractures can be caused by trauma, overuse, or underlying medical conditions.

Motor dysfunction following a fracture can be mild or severe, depending on the extent and location of the fracture. It can affect the ability to move the upper limb, grip objects, or perform daily activities such as dressing or eating. Motor dysfunction may also be accompanied by pain, swelling, and stiffness.

Fractures of the upper limb bones, including the clavicle, scapula, humerus, radius, ulna, and hand bones, can lead to motor dysfunction. The location and type of fracture determine the degree and type of motor dysfunction. For example, a fracture of the humerus near the shoulder joint can affect shoulder movement, while a fracture of the wrist can affect hand and finger movements.

Treatment for upper limb fractures typically involves immobilization of the affected limb using casts or braces to allow for healing. Physical therapy and rehabilitation are often required to restore range of motion, strength, and function of the affected limb.

Overall, upper limb bone fractures and resulting motor dysfunction can have a significant impact on daily activities and quality of life. Early diagnosis, appropriate treatment, and rehabilitation can help minimize the impact of the injury on motor function and promote optimal recovery.

Soft tissue damage

Soft tissue damage and motor dysfunction are common complications of bone fractures and other injuries. Soft tissue damage can occur due to inflammation, swelling, hemorrhage, and nerve injuries. Inflammation of the bursa near the joint is known as bursitis, while inflammation of a muscle attachment is known as tendonitis. These conditions can cause pain and limited mobility of the affected joint.

Bursitis is commonly seen in the shoulder, elbow, hip, and knee joints. It can result in pain, swelling, and limited movement of the joint. The inflammation of the bursa can be caused by repetitive motions, injury, or infection.

Tendonitis is commonly seen in the elbow, wrist, and shoulder joints. It can result in pain, swelling, and restricted movement of the joint. Tendonitis is typically caused by repetitive stress or injury to the affected area.

In some cases, confined movement can be due to inflammation of the muscle or soft tissue surrounding the muscle. This can result in muscle spasms, pain, and limited range of motion.

Fracture of the Olecranon

A fracture of the olecranon is a type of upper limb bone fracture that involves the bony prominence of the ulna at the elbow joint. This type of fracture can be caused by direct trauma to the elbow or by a fall on an outstretched hand. The main symptom of an olecranon fracture is pain and swelling at the elbow, and limited range of motion of the joint.

Motor dysfunction can also occur as a result of an olecranon fracture. This is because the olecranon process serves as an attachment site for the triceps muscle, which is responsible for extending the elbow joint. A fracture of the olecranon can disrupt this attachment site, leading to weakness or inability to extend the elbow.

Treatment of olecranon fracture may involve immobilization of the elbow joint with a cast or brace to allow for healing of the bone. Physical therapy may also be necessary to restore strength and range of motion to the affected joint. In severe cases, surgery may be required to realign and stabilize the fractured bone.

Chapter 9: Upper Limb Motor Dysfunction

Fracture of the distal end of the radius

A fracture of the distal end of the radius, also known as a wrist fracture, is a common injury that can result in motor dysfunction. This type of fracture usually occurs as a result of a fall onto an outstretched hand, which can cause the bone to break at the point where it joins the wrist.

Some common causes of a distal radius fracture include: Falling onto an outstretched hand, Motor vehicle accidents, Sports injuries, and Osteoporosis

Motor dysfunction can occur due to the disruption of the wrist joint and the surrounding soft tissue. Depending on the severity of the fracture, there may be limited mobility and strength in the wrist, making it difficult to perform everyday activities that require wrist movement. Pain and swelling are also common symptoms that can limit the range of motion in the wrist.

In severe cases, surgical intervention may be required to repair the fracture and restore proper function to the wrist joint. Physical therapy may also be recommended to help with the rehabilitation process and to restore strength and mobility to the affected wrist.

Fracture of the distal end of the radius

A fracture of the distal end of the radius is more common in adults over fifty, especially women who may have osteoporosis. The leading cause of the fracture is forced dorsiflexion of the hand, often due to slipping or tripping with the forearm and hand in a pronated position.

After a radius fracture, the distal fragment of the radius is displaced posteriorly, and in about 40% of cases, there is an avulsed ulnar styloid process. The location relationship between the radial and ulnar styloid processes is reversed, resulting in a "dinner fork deformity" in Colles' fracture, which is located about 2 cm from the distal end of the radius (Fig. 9.7).

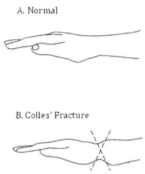

Figure 9.7. The figure shows the appearance of a wrist and forearm with Colles' fracture. Dinner fork deformity is due to the distal fragment of the radius overriding the rest of the bone.

Despite the deformity, the prognosis of a fracture of the distal end of the radius is good because the blood supply to this region is rich, especially in the forearm and wrist regions.

Chapter 9: Upper Limb Motor Dysfunction

Impacted fracture of the humerus surgical neck

An impacted fracture of the surgical neck of the humerus is a common type of fracture in older adults, particularly women, and can result from a variety of mechanisms, such as a fall on an outstretched arm or direct trauma to the shoulder. The surgical neck is a narrowed part of the humerus, located between the greater and lesser tubercles, and it is an area of weakness in the bone.

In an impacted fracture, the bone is compressed, and the fractured ends are wedged into each other. This type of fracture often occurs in older adults because their bones are weaker and more susceptible to compression forces. Impacted fractures of the surgical neck of the humerus can result in pain, swelling, and restricted range of motion of the shoulder joint.

Motor dysfunction can occur as a result of an impacted fracture of the surgical neck of the humerus, particularly in cases where there is displacement of the bone fragments. The deltoid muscle, which attaches to the humerus, may be affected, leading to weakness or paralysis of the shoulder. In addition, the axillary nerve, which runs through the surgical neck of the humerus, may be damaged in cases where the bone fragments are displaced, resulting in motor dysfunction of the deltoid muscle and sensory loss over the shoulder. Physical therapy is often necessary to restore range of motion and strength to the shoulder joint following an impacted fracture of the surgical neck of the humerus. In severe cases, surgery may be required to realign the bone fragments and restore function to the shoulder joint.

Transverse fracture of the body of the humerus

A transverse fracture of the body of the humerus refers to a break in the humerus bone that runs horizontally across the shaft of the bone. This type of fracture can be caused by a variety of factors, including trauma from a fall, a direct blow to the arm, or a sports-related injury.

Symptoms of a transverse fracture of the body of the humerus can include severe pain, swelling, bruising, and difficulty moving the affected arm. In some cases, the arm may appear deformed or misaligned. Numbness or tingling may also be present if the fracture has caused nerve damage.

Treatment for a transverse fracture of the body of the humerus typically involves immobilization of the arm in a cast or brace to allow the bone to heal. In more severe cases, surgery may be required to realign the bone and stabilize it with pins, plates, or screws.

Motor dysfunction can occur as a result of a transverse fracture of the body of the humerus, particularly if the fracture has caused nerve damage. This can lead to weakness, numbness, and a decreased range of motion in the affected arm. Physical therapy and rehabilitation exercises may be recommended to help improve function and mobility in the arm.

Transverse fracture of the body of the humerus

A transverse fracture of the body of the humerus is a break that occurs horizontally across the shaft of the upper arm bone (humerus). This type of fracture can be caused by a variety of things, including a fall onto an outstretched arm, a direct blow to the arm, or a car accident.

In terms of motor dysfunction, a transverse fracture of the humerus can result in significant pain, swelling, and limited range of motion in the affected arm. Depending on the severity of the fracture and any associated nerve or blood vessel damage, the individual may also experience weakness, numbness, or tingling in the affected arm.

In some cases, surgery may be necessary to realign the fractured bone and stabilize it with pins, plates, or screws. Physical therapy is also typically recommended to help restore strength and mobility in the affected arm. With proper treatment and rehabilitation, most individuals with a transverse fracture of the humerus can expect to regain normal function in their arm over time.

Fracture of the Scaphoid Bone

A fracture of the scaphoid bone is a break that occurs in the small bone located near the base of the thumb. This type of fracture is typically caused by a fall onto an outstretched hand, particularly when the hand is extended and the weight of the body is applied to the thumb.

In terms of motor dysfunction, a fracture of the scaphoid bone can result in pain and tenderness in the area of the wrist, particularly when the thumb or wrist is moved. The individual may also experience swelling and limited range of motion in the wrist and hand. Depending on the severity of the fracture and any associated nerve or blood vessel damage, the individual may also experience weakness, numbness, or tingling in the affected hand and fingers.

Because the scaphoid bone has a poor blood supply, healing can be slow and complications may arise if the fracture is not properly treated. Treatment typically involves immobilization of the wrist and hand with a cast or splint to allow the bone to heal. In some cases, surgery may be necessary to realign the fractured bone and stabilize it with pins or screws.

If left untreated or improperly treated, a fracture of the scaphoid bone can result in long-term motor dysfunction, including chronic pain, weakness, and limited range of motion in the affected wrist and hand. Early and appropriate treatment is crucial to minimize the risk of these complications.

Chapter 9: Upper Limb Motor Dysfunction

Snuffbox

The snuffbox is a small triangular depression or hollow located on the radial side of the dorsum (back) of the hand, between the tendons of the extensor pollicis longus and extensor pollicis brevis muscles. It is so named because it was once commonly used for the inhalation of snuff.

The snuffbox is an important anatomical landmark in the wrist and hand, as it is used by healthcare providers to help locate the scaphoid bone, which lies deep within the wrist. Injuries to the scaphoid bone, such as fractures, can cause pain and limited function in the wrist and hand, and identifying the location of the snuffbox can aid in the diagnosis and treatment of these injuries.

Additionally, the snuffbox is an important reference point for anatomical descriptions of the hand and wrist, as many muscles, tendons, nerves, and blood vessels are located nearby. For example, the radial artery, which supplies blood to the hand and fingers, can be palpated within the snuffbox.

Mallet or Baseball Finger

Mallet finger, also known as baseball finger, is an injury that occurs when the extensor tendon of the finger is damaged. This can occur when a ball or other object strikes the tip of the finger, causing the fingertip to be forced downward while the finger is extended. This results in a tear or avulsion of the extensor tendon from its attachment to the bone.

Symptoms of mallet finger include pain, swelling, and inability to fully extend the finger at the end joint. The fingertip may droop and the individual may have difficulty performing fine motor tasks that require the use of the affected finger.

Mallet finger is typically diagnosed through physical examination and X-ray imaging. Treatment may involve immobilization of the finger with a splint or cast for several weeks to allow the tendon to heal. In some cases, surgery may be necessary to repair the damaged tendon.

If left untreated, mallet finger can result in long-term functional deficits, including weakness, stiffness, and decreased range of motion in the affected finger. Therefore, prompt diagnosis and appropriate treatment are important to minimize the risk of complications and optimize recovery.

BURSITIS

Upper limb bursitis is a condition in which the bursae, small fluid-filled sacs that cushion the joints and reduce friction between bones, become inflamed. Bursitis can occur in any joint of the upper limb, including the shoulder, elbow, wrist, and hand.

Symptoms of upper limb bursitis include pain, swelling, and tenderness in the affected joint, as well as limited range of motion

Chapter 9: Upper Limb Motor Dysfunction

and stiffness. In some cases, the inflammation can lead to motor dysfunction, such as weakness or loss of muscle control in the affected limb.

The severity of motor dysfunction in upper limb bursitis depends on the location and extent of the inflammation. For example, bursitis in the shoulder joint can cause weakness and difficulty lifting the arm, while bursitis in the wrist or hand can cause difficulty with grip strength and fine motor tasks.

Treatment of upper limb bursitis typically involves rest, ice, and anti-inflammatory medications to reduce swelling and pain. In more severe cases, a corticosteroid injection may be necessary to alleviate inflammation. Physical therapy and rehabilitation exercises may also be recommended to help restore strength and mobility to the affected limb.

If left untreated, upper limb bursitis can lead to chronic pain and dysfunction, making it important to seek medical attention if you experience persistent symptoms in your upper limb joint.

Subacromial Bursitis

Subacromial bursitis is a condition in which the subacromial bursa, a small fluid-filled sac located between the rotator cuff tendons and the acromion bone in the shoulder, becomes inflamed. This inflammation can cause pain and stiffness in the shoulder, as well as limited range of motion.

In some cases, subacromial bursitis can lead to motor dysfunction, such as weakness or loss of muscle control in the affected shoulder. This can occur due to the pain and inflammation limiting the ability to move the shoulder and use the affected muscles. Over time, this can result in muscle atrophy and further loss of strength.

The severity of motor dysfunction in subacromial bursitis depends on the extent and duration of the inflammation, as well as any underlying conditions that may be contributing to the problem. Treatment of subacromial bursitis typically involves rest, ice, anti-inflammatory medication, and physical therapy to reduce pain and inflammation, restore range of motion, and improve strength and function.

If left untreated, subacromial bursitis can lead to chronic pain, limited mobility, and muscle weakness in the shoulder. It's important to seek medical attention if you are experiencing persistent shoulder pain or stiffness, or if you notice any changes in your shoulder strength or function. Early treatment can help prevent further damage and improve outcomes.

Student's elbow

Student's elbow, also known as olecranon bursitis, is a condition in which the bursa located at the tip of the elbow becomes inflamed and filled with fluid, causing swelling and pain. The condition is often caused by repetitive pressure or trauma to the elbow, such as resting it on a desk for long periods of time.

In some cases, student's elbow can lead to motor dysfunction, such as weakness or loss of muscle control in the affected arm. This can occur due to the pain and inflammation limiting the ability to move the elbow and use the affected muscles. Over time, this can result in muscle atrophy and further loss of strength.

The severity of motor dysfunction in student's elbow depends on the extent and duration of the inflammation, as well as any underlying conditions that may be contributing to the problem. Treatment of student's elbow typically involves rest, ice, anti-inflammatory medication, and physical therapy to reduce pain and inflammation, restore range of motion, and improve strength and function.

Tennis elbow

Tennis elbow, also known as lateral epicondylitis, is a condition in which the outer part of the elbow becomes painful and tender due to overuse or repetitive strain. Despite its name, tennis elbow is not limited to tennis players and can affect anyone who engages in activities that involve repetitive motion of the wrist and forearm.

In addition to pain and tenderness, tennis elbow can lead to motor dysfunction, such as weakness or loss of muscle control in the affected arm. This can occur due to the pain and inflammation limiting the ability to move the wrist and use the affected muscles. Over time, this can result in muscle atrophy and further loss of strength.

The severity of motor dysfunction in tennis elbow depends on the extent and duration of the inflammation. Treatment of tennis elbow typically involves rest, ice, anti-inflammatory medication, and physical therapy to reduce pain and inflammation, restore range of motion, and improve strength and function.

Carpal Tunnel Syndrome

Carpal tunnel syndrome refers to a condition characterized by increased pressure inside the carpal tunnel, a narrow passageway located in the wrist, between the bones and flexor retinaculum. This compression can result from various causes, such as infection, fluid retention, or repetitive hand movements leading to swelling of the tendons or synovial sheaths.

The median nerve, which runs through the carpal tunnel, provides sensation to the lateral three and a half digits and controls the movement of the thumb through its motor branch. Thus, compression of the median nerve can cause symptoms such as abnormal or loss of sensation in the affected fingers, weakness in the thumb, and difficulty performing daily tasks that require grip strength.

Chapter 9: Upper Limb Motor Dysfunction

As carpal tunnel syndrome progresses, motor and sensory abnormalities become more prominent, and patients may experience difficulty with tasks such as buttoning a shirt or holding objects. To alleviate symptoms, surgical intervention, such as a flexor retinaculum release, may be necessary.

Therefore, carpal tunnel syndrome is caused by increased pressure within the carpal tunnel, leading to compression of the median nerve and resulting in motor and sensory dysfunction in the hand and wrist.

Raynaud's Phenomenon

Raynaud's phenomenon is a condition in which the blood vessels in the fingers and toes constrict excessively in response to cold temperatures or emotional stress, causing the affected areas to turn white or blue and feel cold and numb. This constriction of the blood vessels reduces blood flow to the fingers and toes, leading to the characteristic symptoms.

The cause of Raynaud's phenomenon is not fully understood, but it is believed to be related to abnormalities in the nervous system controlling blood vessel constriction and dilation, as well as abnormalities in the blood vessels themselves.

Treatment of Raynaud's phenomenon depends on the severity of the symptoms and the underlying cause. In mild cases, simply avoiding triggers such as cold temperatures and stress may be enough to prevent symptoms. In more severe cases, medications that improve blood flow, such as calcium channel blockers or alpha blockers, may be prescribed.

CHAPTER 10 LOWER LIMB MOTOR DYSFUNCTION

Lower limb motor dysfunction refers to a condition in which there is a decrease in the normal functioning of the muscles, nerves, and other structures that control movement in the legs and feet. This can be caused by a variety of factors, including neurological disorders, injuries, infections, and certain medications.

Some of the common symptoms of lower limb motor dysfunction include difficulty walking or standing, weakness or numbness in the legs, cramps or spasms, and difficulty with balance and coordination. Depending on the underlying cause, other symptoms may also be present, such as pain, swelling, or changes in sensation.

Hip region

Hip region motor dysfunction refers to a condition where there is a decrease in the normal functioning of the muscles, nerves, and other structures that control movement in the hip and surrounding area. This can be caused by a variety of factors, including neurological disorders, injuries, infections, and certain medications.

Some common symptoms of hip region motor dysfunction include difficulty walking or standing, weakness or numbness in the hip or surrounding area, cramps or spasms, and difficulty with balance and coordination. Depending on the underlying cause, other symptoms may also be present, such as pain, swelling, or changes in sensation.

Hip joint movement

The hip joint is a ball-and-socket joint that connects the femur to the pelvis. It allows for a wide range of movement, including flexion, extension, abduction, adduction, internal rotation, and external rotation. These movements are controlled by the major muscles involved in hip movement, including the hip flexors, hip extensors, hip abductors, hip adductors, and hip rotators.

1. The hip flexors, including the iliopsoas, rectus femoris, sartorius, and pectineus muscles, are responsible for hip flexion.
2. Hip extension is primarily controlled by the hamstrings and gluteus maximus muscles, which are innervated by the sciatic nerve.
3. The gluteus medius and gluteus minimus muscles, innervated by the superior gluteal nerve, work together to abduct the hip joint.

Hip dysfunction: Dysfunction in the hip joint can result in conditions such as hip osteoarthritis, hip bursitis, hip labral tears, hip impingement syndrome, and hip fractures. These conditions can cause pain, stiffness, weakness, and limited range of motion in the hip joint, affecting the patient's ability to perform daily activities. Management of hip dysfunction may involve manual therapy, stretching, strengthening exercises, and other modalities.

Sciatic nerve injury

The sciatic nerve is the largest nerve in the body, and it originates from the lower spine and travels through the pelvis, buttocks, and down the back of each leg. It provides sensation to the skin of the leg and foot, and it controls the muscles in the back of the thigh, lower leg, and foot.

Sciatic nerve injury can occur due to a variety of reasons, such as compression of the nerve, hip joint dislocation, fracture of the neck of the femur, buttock injection, and lumbar-sacral joint injury. One of the most common causes of sciatic nerve injury is piriformis syndrome, where the sciatic nerve is compressed by the piriformis muscle, which is located in the buttock region.

The symptoms of sciatic nerve injury typically include pain, which is called sciatica. The pain is experienced in the gluteal region, the posterior aspect of the thigh, the posterior and lateral aspects of the leg, and the lateral aspects of the ankle and foot. In addition to pain, other symptoms may include weakness, numbness, or tingling in the affected leg or foot. Motor dysfunction may also be displayed when the ankle reflex disappears.

In addition, it's worth noting that the sciatic nerve does not directly supply the muscles and joints in the gluteal region, but rather innervates the muscles and joints of the lower limbs. Sciatica, the pain caused by sciatic nerve injury, can be due to various causes such as spinal stenosis or a herniated disc, and treatment will depend on the specific underlying condition.

Treatment for sciatic nerve injury depends on the underlying cause of the injury. Conservative treatments, such as rest, ice, and anti-inflammatory medications, may be effective in relieving pain and reducing inflammation. Physical therapy, stretching exercises, and other rehabilitation techniques may also be recommended to improve mobility and strength in the affected leg. In some cases, surgical intervention may be necessary to relieve pressure on the nerve and restore function.

Hip Joint Dislocation

The hip joint is a ball-and-socket joint consisting of the head of the femur and the acetabulum of the hip bone. The capsule of the hip joint is composed of strong fibrous tissue, and it contains several ligaments, including the iliofemoral ligament, pubofemoral ligament, ischiofemoral ligament, and the ligament of the femoral head. The artery at the head of the femur travels inside the ligament of the ligament of the femoral head and is the primary source of blood supply to the femur. If it is damaged during hip joint dislocation, recovery becomes difficult.

Hip joint dislocation can be caused by various factors, including car accidents where the knee strikes the dashboard, congenital deficiency of the acetabular rim, or a sports injury. Posterior dislocation of the head of the femur is the most common pathology of hip joint dislocation. This is because the head of the femur moves out of the hip joint posteriorly, often damaging the posterior margin of the acetabulum and acetabular labrum, as well as the articular capsule of the hip joint. In some cases, the artery at the head of the femur may also be torn, leading to necrosis of the head of the femur.

Symptoms of hip joint dislocation include pain, a flexed hip joint, an adducted and medially rotated thigh, and a shortened leg due to the hip muscles pulling the femur upward after the dislocation. If the sciatic nerve is severely injured, the leg may be paralyzed.

Diagnosis of hip joint dislocation is based on the patient's history, symptoms, and an X-ray examination. The X-ray will show displacement of the bones. Prompt medical attention is necessary to ensure the best possible outcome, and treatment may involve reduction of the dislocation, pain management, physical therapy, or even surgery in severe cases.

Fracture of the Neck of the Femur

Fracture of the neck of the femur, also known as a hip fracture, is a common injury in elderly people. The femoral neck is the region between the femoral head and the greater trochanter of the femur bone.

Causes: Hip fractures are commonly caused by falls in elderly people with weakened bones due to osteoporosis or other bone diseases. Other causes include trauma, such as car accidents or sports injuries, and pathological fractures due to cancer or other underlying medical conditions.

Motor Dysfunction: Hip fractures often result in significant motor dysfunction. The patient may have severe pain and an inability to bear weight on the affected leg. The leg may appear shortened, externally rotated, and abducted. Fracture displacement can result in muscle spasm, causing muscle weakness and joint stiffness. In addition, the patient may experience nerve damage, leading to numbness, tingling, or weakness in the affected leg.

The femoral neck is an area of high mechanical stress, and its blood supply is susceptible to disruption after a fracture. The blood supply to the femoral head passes through the neck, and fracture displacement can cause interruption of the blood flow, leading to avascular necrosis of the femoral head. The compromised blood supply also impedes fracture healing, making hip fractures difficult to treat and often requiring surgical intervention. The resulting pain, motor dysfunction, and other complications can significantly impact the patient's mobility and quality of life.

KNEE REGION

Motor dysfunction in the knee region can occur due to various reasons, such as nerve injury or damage to the muscles, bones, or joints. Common causes of motor dysfunction in the knee region include knee joint injuries, such as ligament tears or patellar dislocation, nerve injuries like common peroneal nerve injury or femoral nerve injury, and conditions like osteoarthritis and rheumatoid arthritis.

Symptoms of motor dysfunction in the knee region can include weakness or inability to move the knee joint, difficulty walking, and problems with balance and coordination. Treatment for motor dysfunction in the knee region depends on the underlying cause and may include physical therapy, medication, or surgery.

Knee joint movement

The knee joint is a complex hinge joint that connects the thigh bone (femur) and the shin bone (tibia). It is responsible for bearing weight and allowing movements such as flexion, extension, rotation, and stability of the lower leg.

Knee Joint Movements:

- Flexion: bending the knee joint
- Extension: straightening the knee joint
- Rotation: internal and external rotation of the knee joint
- Stability: providing stability during weight-bearing activities

Knee Joint Muscles:

- Quadriceps femoris: a group of four muscles located in the front of the thigh that are responsible for knee extension
- Hamstrings: a group of three muscles located in the back of the thigh that are responsible for knee flexion
- Gastrocnemius: a calf muscle that crosses the knee joint and assists with knee flexion
- Popliteus: a small muscle located at the back of the knee joint that assists with knee rotation and stability

Knee Joint Dysfunctions:

- Knee ligament injuries: can occur due to trauma or overuse and result in pain, instability, and limited range of motion
- Meniscus tears: the meniscus is a cartilage structure that cushions the knee joint, and tears can cause pain, swelling, and reduced range of motion

- Patellofemoral syndrome: a condition in which the patella (kneecap) does not track properly over the femur, causing pain and discomfort during activities that involve bending and straightening the knee

- Osteoarthritis: a degenerative joint disease that can cause pain, stiffness, and reduced range of motion in the knee joint

- Patellar tendonitis: an overuse injury that can cause pain and inflammation in the patellar tendon, which connects the patella to the tibia.

Ageing related knee injuries

As the human body ages, the knee joint undergoes degenerative changes that increase the risk of injury. Some common knee injuries associated with aging include:

1. Osteoarthritis: This is the most common type of arthritis that affects the knee joint. It occurs due to the degeneration of the cartilage that cushions the ends of the bones in the joint, leading to pain, stiffness, and reduced mobility.

2. Meniscal tears: The menisci are cartilage pads that act as shock absorbers in the knee joint. As the knee ages, these pads can become more brittle and prone to tearing, especially during physical activity or sudden twisting movements.

3. Tendinitis: Tendons are fibrous bands that connect muscles to bones. Overuse or age-related degeneration can lead to tendinitis, which is inflammation of the tendons around the knee joint. This can cause pain and swelling, and can limit the range of motion of the joint.

4. Bursitis: Bursae are small fluid-filled sacs that cushion and lubricate the knee joint. As the knee ages, these sacs can become inflamed and swollen, leading to pain and reduced mobility.

5. Ligament injuries: The ligaments in the knee joint, such as the ACL and MCL, can become weaker and more prone to injury as the knee ages. Sports and physical activity can also increase the risk of ligament tears.

Preventative measures, such as maintaining a healthy weight, staying physically active, and wearing appropriate footwear, can help reduce the risk of knee injuries associated with aging.

Sports related knee injuries

Sports are a common cause of knee ligament injuries, which can occur due to direct blows, sudden changes in direction, twisting, or hyperextension of the knee joint. The knee joint is a complex hinge joint that is stabilized by four major ligaments: the anterior cruciate ligament (ACL), posterior cruciate ligament (PCL), medial collateral ligament (MCL), and lateral collateral ligament (LCL).

- ACL injuries are one of the most common knee ligament injuries in sports, especially in sports that involve cutting, pivoting, and jumping, such as basketball, football, and soccer. ACL injuries often occur when the knee is forced to twist or rotate suddenly, causing the ACL to tear. This can happen when the foot is planted on the ground and the body is forced to rotate or when the knee is hyperextended.
- PCL injuries are less common than ACL injuries and often occur due to direct blows to the front of the knee, such as in a car accident or a fall on a bent knee. PCL injuries can also occur during sports that involve falls, such as skiing or football.
- MCL injuries are common in sports that involve contact, such as football or rugby. MCL injuries often occur due to a blow to the outer part of the knee, causing the MCL to stretch or tear.
- LCL injuries are less common than MCL injuries and often occur due to a blow to the inner part of the knee, causing the LCL to stretch or tear.

Knee ligament injuries can be serious and may require surgery and extensive rehabilitation to recover fully. Proper conditioning, technique, and protective gear can help prevent knee ligament injuries in sports.

Common Fibular Nerve Injury

The common fibular nerve is a branch of the sciatic nerve that runs along the medial side of the biceps femoris muscle and its tendon, passing over the posterior aspect of the head of the fibula and winding around the neck of the fibula to the fibularis longus muscle. It supplies the skin of the lateral part of the posterior aspect of the leg, the knee joint, and the muscles of the anterior and lateral compartments of the leg and dorsum of the foot.

Causes: Injury to the common fibular nerve is often a complication of lower limb injuries because this nerve winds superficially around the fibular neck. It is commonly seen in fractures at the fibular neck, but can also occur when the knee joint is injured or dislocated.

Symptoms: Common symptoms of common fibular nerve injury include both sensory and motor abnormalities. The motor component is characterized by paralysis of all the muscles in the anterior and lateral compartments of the leg, including the dorsiflexors of the ankle and evertors of the foot. As a result, the patient may experience foot drop, which is a gait abnormality characterized by dragging the toes on the floor when walking, also known as "steppage gait." (Fig. 10.1) There is also a loss of sensation in the anterolateral aspect of the leg and the dorsal aspect of the foot.

Chapter 10 Lower Limb Motor Dysfunction

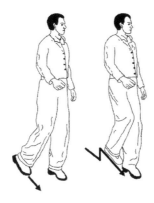

Figure 10.1. Steppage gait caused by common fibular nerve injury subject (right), and healthy subject (left**).**

Knee joint injury

The knee joint is susceptible to various types of injuries due to its complex anatomy and the significant stresses it endures during physical activity. Some common knee injuries include:

1. ACL tear: The anterior cruciate ligament (ACL) is a crucial stabilizing ligament in the knee joint. ACL tears are common in sports that involve sudden stops, changes in direction, or jumping. Symptoms of an ACL tear include pain, swelling, instability, and difficulty bearing weight.

2. Meniscus tear: The meniscus is a piece of cartilage that cushions the knee joint. Meniscus tears are often caused by twisting or rotating the knee while bearing weight. Symptoms include pain, swelling, stiffness, and difficulty straightening the knee.

3. Patellar tendinitis: Also known as jumper's knee, patellar tendinitis is an overuse injury that affects the patellar tendon, which connects the kneecap to the shinbone. It is common in sports that involve jumping, such as basketball and volleyball. Symptoms include pain and swelling below the kneecap.

4. Patellar dislocation: A patellar dislocation occurs when the kneecap slips out of place, usually towards the outside of the knee. It can be caused by a sudden change in direction or a direct blow to the knee. Symptoms include pain, swelling, instability, and difficulty bending or straightening the knee.

5. MCL tear: The medial collateral ligament (MCL) is a band of tissue on the inside of the knee that provides stability. MCL tears are often caused by a direct blow to the outside of the knee or a twisting injury. Symptoms include pain, swelling, and instability.

Treatment for knee injuries depends on the severity and type of injury. It can include rest, ice, compression, elevation, physical therapy, and surgery in some cases. Prevention measures, such as proper warm-up and stretching before physical activity and using proper technique during sports, can help reduce the risk of knee injuries.

Lachman's Test

Lachman's test is a physical examination maneuver used to assess the integrity of the anterior cruciate ligament (ACL) in the knee joint. The ACL is a ligament that runs diagonally through the middle of the knee joint and helps stabilize the knee during movement.

During the Lachman's test, the patient lies on their back with their knee flexed to about 20-30 degrees. The examiner stabilizes the patient's thigh with one hand while pulling the lower leg forward with the other hand. The examiner then assesses the amount of anterior translation of the tibia relative to the femur.

If there is excessive anterior tibial translation and a lack of a firm endpoint, it may indicate a torn ACL. A firm endpoint indicates a healthy ACL. This test is considered one of the most reliable tests for diagnosing an ACL injury, with a sensitivity of over 85% and a specificity of over 90%.

ANKLE REGION

The ankle region refers to the joint that connects the foot and leg bones. It is comprised of three bones: the tibia, fibula, and talus. The tibia and fibula bones of the leg come together to form a mortise joint, which the talus bone fits into. The ankle region is responsible for supporting the weight of the body and enabling movement of the foot.

The ankle region is surrounded by several ligaments that provide stability to the joint. These include the medial and lateral collateral ligaments, the anterior and posterior talofibular ligaments, and the calcaneofibular ligament.

The muscles of the ankle region are responsible for controlling the movement of the foot and ankle joint. The muscles that move the ankle joint are divided into three compartments: the anterior compartment, the lateral compartment, and the posterior compartment. The anterior compartment includes the tibialis anterior and extensor hallucis longus muscles, which are responsible for dorsiflexion (lifting the foot upwards). The lateral compartment includes the peroneus longus and peroneus brevis muscles, which are responsible for eversion (turning the foot outwards). The posterior compartment includes the gastrocnemius, soleus, and plantaris muscles, which are responsible for plantarflexion (pointing the foot downwards).

Injuries to the ankle region are common, with ankle sprains being one of the most common injuries. Ankle sprains occur when the ligaments in the ankle are stretched or torn, usually due to a sudden twisting or turning motion. Ankle fractures and dislocations are also possible, and can result from high-impact injuries such as falls or sports-related collisions.

Ankle injury associated with sports

Ankle injuries are common in many sports, particularly those that involve running, jumping, and quick changes of direction. Some of the most common sports associated with ankle injuries include basketball, soccer, football, and volleyball.

The most common type of ankle injury is an ankle sprain, which occurs when the ligaments that hold the ankle bones in place are stretched or torn. This can happen when the foot twists or turns suddenly, such as when an athlete lands awkwardly or changes direction abruptly. Ankle sprains can range from mild to severe, depending on the extent of the ligament damage.

Another common ankle injury in sports is an ankle fracture, which occurs when one or more of the ankle bones are broken. This can happen as a result of a hard impact, such as a fall or collision, or from twisting the ankle too far.

Athletes may also experience Achilles tendon injuries, which occur when the tendon that connects the calf muscles to the heel bone is strained or torn. This can happen when the athlete pushes off forcefully, such as when sprinting or jumping.

The risk of ankle injuries in sports can be influenced by several factors, including the type of sport, playing surface, and athlete's level of conditioning. For example, sports that involve a lot of jumping and landing, such as basketball and volleyball, may increase the risk of ankle sprains. Playing on uneven or slippery surfaces can also increase the risk of ankle injuries. Athletes who have poor ankle strength, flexibility, and balance may be more prone to ankle injuries.

Preventing ankle injuries in sports can involve measures such as proper conditioning, warm-up exercises, wearing appropriate footwear, and using ankle braces or supports. Athletes should also be aware of their movements and take steps to avoid putting excessive stress on the ankle joint. In cases where an ankle injury does occur, prompt treatment and rehabilitation can help reduce pain, swelling, and stiffness, and speed up recovery.

Ankle injuries associated with ageing

As we age, the bones and soft tissues in our body can become weaker and more fragile, which can increase the risk of ankle injuries. Some common ankle injuries associated with aging include:

1. Ankle sprains: As we age, the ligaments that support the ankle joint may become weaker and less elastic, making them more susceptible to sprains. Ankle sprains occur when the ankle is twisted or turned beyond its normal range of motion, causing the ligaments to stretch or tear.

2. Achilles tendon injuries: The Achilles tendon is a thick, fibrous band of tissue that connects the calf muscles to the heel bone. As we age, the Achilles tendon can become less flexible and

more prone to injury. Achilles tendon injuries can range from mild strains to complete tears.

3. Osteoarthritis: Osteoarthritis is a degenerative joint disease that can affect the ankle joint. It occurs when the protective cartilage on the ends of the bones wears down over time, leading to pain, stiffness, and swelling in the ankle joint.

4. Gout: Gout is a type of arthritis that can affect the ankle joint. It occurs when there is a buildup of uric acid crystals in the joint, leading to sudden and severe pain, swelling, and redness.

5. Fractures: As we age, our bones become more brittle and prone to fractures. Ankle fractures can occur as a result of a fall or other trauma, or as a result of osteoporosis, a condition that causes bones to become weak and brittle.

Overall, ankle injuries associated with aging are caused by a combination of factors, including changes in bone and soft tissue structure, decreased flexibility and mobility, and a higher risk of falls and other accidents. Maintaining a healthy lifestyle, including regular exercise and a balanced diet, can help reduce the risk of ankle injuries and promote overall joint health as we age.

Ankle joint dysfunction

Ankle joint dysfunction refers to any impairment in the normal functioning of the ankle joint. The ankle joint is composed of the lower ends of the tibia and fibula (the two bones in the lower leg) and the talus bone (a bone in the foot). The ankle joint allows for movement of the foot in multiple directions, such as plantar flexion (pointing the foot downward), dorsiflexion (lifting the foot upward), inversion (turning the foot inward), and eversion (turning the foot outward).

Ankle joint dysfunction can be caused by a variety of factors, including:

1. Sprains: An ankle sprain is a common injury in which the ligaments connecting the bones in the ankle joint are stretched or torn, often due to excessive twisting or rolling of the ankle.

2. Fractures: Ankle fractures can occur as a result of a traumatic injury, such as a fall or a car accident.

3. Arthritis: Arthritis is a degenerative joint disease that can affect the ankle joint, leading to pain, stiffness, and limited range of motion.

4. Tendinitis: Tendinitis is an inflammation of the tendons that attach the muscles to the bones in the ankle joint, often due to overuse or repetitive stress.

5. Nerve damage: Damage to the nerves that supply the ankle joint can lead to numbness, tingling, and weakness in the foot and ankle.

Symptoms of ankle joint dysfunction can include pain, swelling, stiffness, difficulty walking or bearing weight on the affected foot, and instability or weakness in the ankle. Treatment for ankle joint dysfunction depends on the underlying cause and can include rest, ice, compression, elevation, physical therapy, medication, or surgery.

Pott's Fracture

Pott's fracture, also known as a bimalleolar ankle fracture, is a type of ankle fracture that involves the distal fibula and tibia bones. It occurs when there is an external rotation of the foot, along with an inward displacement of the ankle joint. This can happen as a result of a fall or a sudden twisting motion, which can cause the ankle to become unstable and lead to a fracture.

Pott's fracture is more common in older adults due to age-related changes in bone density, decreased muscle strength, and balance issues. In addition, older adults may have other medical conditions that can affect their bone health, such as osteoporosis or arthritis. As a result, they may be more susceptible to fractures from falls or other accidents.

Symptoms of Pott's fracture may include pain, swelling, bruising, and difficulty walking or bearing weight on the affected ankle. Treatment typically involves immobilization of the ankle with a cast or boot, and in some cases, surgery may be necessary to realign and stabilize the fractured bones. Rehabilitation and physical therapy may also be necessary to restore range of motion and strength in the ankle.

Sprained Ankle

A sprained ankle is an injury that occurs when the ligaments that support the ankle joint are stretched or torn, usually due to a sudden twisting or turning of the ankle. It is a common injury, especially among athletes and people who engage in physical activities that involve jumping, running, or sudden changes of direction.

The severity of a sprained ankle can vary depending on the extent of the ligament damage. There are three grades of ankle sprains:

1. Grade 1: Mild sprain that involves stretching or slight tearing of the ligament without joint instability.

2. Grade 2: Moderate sprain that involves partial tearing of the ligament with some joint instability.

3. Grade 3: Severe sprain that involves complete tearing of the ligament with significant joint instability.

Symptoms of a sprained ankle include pain, swelling, bruising, and difficulty walking or putting weight on the affected foot. Treatment for a sprained ankle typically involves rest, ice, compression, and elevation of the affected foot to reduce swelling and pain. In some cases, a brace or cast may be needed to immobilize the ankle and promote healing. Physical therapy may also be recommended to help restore range of motion, strength, and stability to the affected ankle.

CHAPTER 11: VERTEBRAL COLUMN INJURY

Introduction

Injuries to the vertebral column, or spine, can be serious and even life-threatening. The vertebral column is composed of 33 individual bones, called vertebrae, which are stacked on top of each other and separated by intervertebral discs. The vertebral column serves to protect the spinal cord, support the body's weight, and allow for movement.

There are many types of injuries that can occur to the vertebral column, including:

1. Fractures: Fractures can occur in any of the individual vertebrae. They can be caused by trauma, such as a fall or car accident, or by medical conditions that weaken the bones, such as osteoporosis.

2. Dislocations: Dislocations occur when the bones of the spine are forced out of their normal position. This can be caused by trauma, such as a fall or car accident.

3. Herniated discs: A herniated disc occurs when the soft inner material of a disc pushes out through a crack in the tough outer layer of the disc. This can put pressure on the spinal cord or nerves, causing pain, numbness, or weakness.

4. Spinal cord injuries: Spinal cord injuries can result from trauma, such as a fall or car accident, or from medical conditions such as tumors or infections. These injuries can cause paralysis, loss of sensation, or other neurological problems.

Symptoms of vertebral column injuries can vary depending on the location and severity of the injury. Common symptoms may include pain, numbness or tingling, weakness, difficulty walking, and loss of bowel or bladder control.

Treatment for vertebral column injuries will depend on the type and severity of the injury. Treatment options may include rest, physical therapy, medications, or surgery. In some cases, a brace or other device may be needed to support the spine during healing. Rehabilitation may also be necessary to help restore function and mobility after an injury.

Motor symptoms caused by vertebral column injury

Motor dysfunction resulting from a vertebral column injury can range from mild to severe, depending on the location and extent of the injury. The motor dysfunction may be temporary or permanent

Chapter 11: Vertebral Column Injury

and can include weakness, paralysis, spasticity, abnormal movements, and changes in coordination and balance.

Injuries to the vertebral column, which includes the bones of the spine, can cause various motor dysfunctions, depending on the location and severity of the injury.

Injuries to the cervical spine (neck) can result in quadriplegia or tetraplegia, while injuries to the thoracic or lumbar spine (mid and lower back) can result in paraplegia.

Here are some common motor dysfunctions caused by vertebral column injury:

1. Paralysis: Severe injuries to the cervical (neck) region of the vertebral column can cause paralysis of the arms, legs, and/or torso. Paralysis occurs when the spinal cord is damaged and can no longer send signals to the muscles.
2. Paresis: Paresis is a partial paralysis or weakness of the limbs or trunk. This can occur with injuries to the thoracic or lumbar regions of the vertebral column.
3. Muscle spasms: Vertebral column injuries can also cause muscle spasms or involuntary muscle contractions. These can be painful and can interfere with movement and daily activities.
4. Abnormal reflexes: Injuries to the vertebral column can also cause abnormal reflexes, such as hyperreflexia (exaggerated reflexes) or hyporeflexia (diminished reflexes).

5. Loss of sensation: Injuries to the vertebral column can cause loss of sensation, such as the ability to feel touch, pressure, or temperature, in the affected areas of the body.
6. Other symptoms: In addition to motor dysfunction, vertebral column injuries can also cause a range of other symptoms, such as loss of sensation, difficulty breathing, bowel or bladder dysfunction, and changes in sexual function.

Treatment of vertebral column injury

Treatment for motor dysfunctions caused by vertebral column injury will depend on the location and severity of the injury, as well as the specific motor dysfunctions present.

Treatment may include immobilization of the affected area, physical therapy, medications to manage pain and muscle spasms, or surgery to stabilize the spine or repair damaged nerves. In some cases, assistive devices such as braces or wheelchairs may also be necessary to help individuals with vertebral column injuries regain mobility and independence.

1. Rehabilitation: Rehabilitation for a vertebral column injury is an essential part of the recovery process. The type and extent of rehabilitation will depend on the severity of the injury and the individual's specific needs and goals. The rehabilitation process typically involves a multidisciplinary team of healthcare professionals, including physicians, physical therapists,

occupational therapists, and other specialists as needed. The goals of rehabilitation for a vertebral column injury may include: 1) Reducing pain and inflammation, 2) Preventing further damage to the spine and spinal cord, 3) Restoring motor function and mobility, 4) Maximizing independence and quality of life, and 5)Providing emotional and psychological support to the individual and their family.

2. Physical therapy: Physical therapy is often the primary focus of rehabilitation, and may include exercises to improve strength, flexibility, balance, and coordination.

3. Occupational therapy: Occupational therapists work with individuals to help them develop the skills and strategies necessary to perform daily activities, such as dressing, grooming, and household tasks, despite any limitations or disabilities resulting from the injury.

Table of some common types of vertebral column injuries

Type of Injury	Description	Motor Dysfunction
Spinal Fracture	A break in one or more vertebrae	Paralysis, paresis, abnormal reflexes
Spinal Cord Injury	Damage to the spinal cord resulting in loss of function	Paralysis, paresis, abnormal reflexes
Herniated Disc	A ruptured or bulging disc that compresses the spinal nerves	Weakness, numbness, tingling, muscle spasms
Spinal Stenosis	Narrowing of the spinal canal that compresses the spinal nerves	Weakness, numbness, tingling, loss of balance
Spondylolisthesis	A vertebra that slips out of place and compresses the nerves	Weakness, numbness, tingling, loss of balance
Vertebral Dislocation	A dislocation or misalignment of one or more vertebrae	Paralysis, paresis, abnormal reflexes, pain

It's important to note that the motor dysfunction caused by these injuries can vary depending on the severity and location of the injury. It's also possible to experience other symptoms, such as pain, loss of sensation, and difficulty with coordination or balance. Treatment for vertebral column injuries will depend on the specific type of injury and the severity of symptoms, but may include rest, physical therapy, medication, or surgery.

Chapter 11: Vertebral Column Injury

CERVICAL VERTEBRAE

Cervical vertebral injury

Cervical vertebrae injuries are injuries that affect the seven vertebrae in the neck region of the spine. Some common cervical vertebrae injuries and their symptoms are:

1. Whiplash injury: This is a common injury caused by sudden and forceful backward and forward movements of the neck, commonly seen in car accidents. Symptoms may include neck pain, stiffness, headaches, dizziness, and blurred vision.

2. Cervical fracture: This is a break in one or more of the cervical vertebrae. Symptoms may include neck pain, stiffness, loss of sensation in arms or legs, difficulty breathing, and paralysis.

3. Cervical dislocation: This is when the vertebrae are displaced from their normal position. Symptoms may include neck pain, stiffness, tingling or numbness in the arms or legs, and weakness.

4. Herniated disc: This is when the soft, gel-like center of a spinal disc pushes out through a tear in the disc's outer layer, putting pressure on surrounding nerves. Symptoms may include neck pain, tingling or numbness in the arms or legs, and weakness.

5. Spinal cord injury: This is a serious injury that can result from any of the above injuries or other trauma to the neck. Symptoms may include loss of sensation or movement in the arms or legs, difficulty breathing, and paralysis.

It's important to seek medical attention immediately if you suspect a cervical vertebrae injury, as prompt treatment can help prevent further damage and improve outcomes.

LUMBAR VERTEBRAE

Lumbar Injury

The lumbar spine is the lower back region of the spine, consisting of five vertebrae. Common lumbar injuries and their symptoms are:

1. Lumbar strain: This is a common injury that occurs when the muscles and ligaments in the lower back are stretched or torn. Symptoms may include low back pain, muscle spasms, and stiffness.

2. Herniated disc: This is when the soft, gel-like center of a spinal disc pushes out through a tear in the disc's outer layer, putting pressure on surrounding nerves. Symptoms may include low back pain, leg pain or numbness, and muscle weakness.

3. Sciatica: This is a condition that occurs when the sciatic nerve, which runs from the lower back down to the legs, is compressed or irritated. Symptoms may include low back pain, leg pain or numbness, and muscle weakness.

4. Spinal stenosis: This is a condition that occurs when the spinal canal narrows, putting pressure on the spinal cord and nerves.

Chapter 11: Vertebral Column Injury

Symptoms may include low back pain, leg pain or numbness, and difficulty standing or walking.

5. Spondylolisthesis: This is a condition that occurs when one vertebra slips out of place onto the vertebra below it. Symptoms may include low back pain, muscle spasms, and stiffness.

It's important to seek medical attention if you suspect a lumbar injury, as prompt treatment can help prevent further damage and improve outcomes.

Table: Common types of lower back injuries

Type of Injury	Description	Motor Dysfunction
Lumbar Strain	A stretching or tearing of the muscles or tendons in the lower back	Muscle spasms, weakness, limited mobility
Lumbar Sprain	A stretching or tearing of the ligaments in the lower back	Muscle spasms, weakness, limited mobility
Herniated Disc	A ruptured or bulging disc that compresses the spinal nerves	Weakness, numbness, tingling, muscle spasms
Spinal Stenosis	Narrowing of the spinal canal that compresses the spinal nerves	Weakness, numbness, tingling, loss of balance
Spondylolisthesis	A vertebra that slips out of place and compresses the nerves	Weakness, numbness, tingling, loss of balance
Sciatica	Compression or irritation of the sciatic nerve	Weakness, numbness, tingling, loss of reflexes

Lower back pain

Lower back pain is a common condition that affects a significant portion of the population. It refers to pain that occurs in the lumbar region, which is the lower part of the spine that consists of five vertebrae (L1-L5). Lower back pain can be acute or chronic, and it can range from mild to severe.

Causes of lower back pain can vary, and they include muscle or ligament strains, herniated discs, sciatica, spinal stenosis, osteoarthritis, and degenerative disc disease. Other risk factors for lower back pain include poor posture, obesity, lack of exercise, and age-related changes in the spine.

Symptoms of lower back pain may include a dull ache, sharp pain, or burning sensation in the lower back, difficulty moving, stiffness, and muscle spasms. In some cases, lower back pain may radiate to the buttocks or legs, indicating nerve involvement.

Treatment for lower back pain depends on the underlying cause and the severity of the condition. Conservative treatment options include rest, ice or heat therapy, over-the-counter pain medications, physical therapy, and chiropractic care. In more severe cases, surgery may be necessary.

Prevention of lower back pain involves maintaining a healthy weight, engaging in regular exercise, practicing good posture, using proper lifting techniques, and avoiding prolonged periods of sitting or standing.

Herniation of nucleus pulposus

A herniation of the nucleus pulposus, also known as a herniated disc, is a condition where the soft, gel-like center of a spinal disc pushes out through a tear in the disc's outer layer, putting pressure on surrounding nerves (Fig. 11.1). This can cause a variety of symptoms, including:

1. Pain: The most common symptom of a herniated disc is pain, which can be felt in the back, neck, arms, or legs, depending on where the herniation is located.

2. Numbness or tingling: Pressure on the nerves can cause numbness or tingling sensations in the arms, legs, or other parts of the body.

3. Weakness: In some cases, a herniated disc can cause weakness in the muscles of the arms, legs, or other affected areas.

4. Loss of bladder or bowel control: In rare cases, a large herniation can put pressure on the nerves that control bladder and bowel function, leading to incontinence.

The causes of a herniated disc can vary, but some common risk factors include:

1. Age: As we age, the discs in our spine can become less flexible and more prone to injury.

2. Trauma: A sudden injury or trauma, such as a fall or car accident, can cause a herniated disc.

3. Repetitive motions: Repeatedly performing the same motions, such as twisting or lifting, can put strain on the spine and increase the risk of a herniated disc.

4. Genetics: Some people may be more predisposed to developing herniated discs due to their genetic makeup.

Treatment for a herniated disc may include rest, physical therapy, pain medication, and in severe cases, surgery. It's important to see a healthcare provider if you experience symptoms of a herniated disc to receive an accurate diagnosis and appropriate treatment.

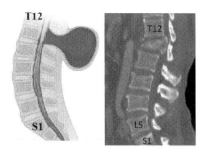

Figure 11.1. Vertebral lumbar injury causing the nucleus pulposus to burst through the annulus fibrosus between T12 and L1. The protruded material can press on or chemically irritate the nerve roots, such as the sciatic nerve roots. Hemorrhage and edema can also be seen.

CHAPTER 12: METHODS FOR DIAGNOSING AND ASSESSING MOTOR DYSFUNCTION

Diagnosis and assessment of motor dysfunction are essential in identifying and characterizing movement disorders, determining the severity of the condition, and developing appropriate treatment plans.

Methods

Here are some of the different methods for diagnosing and assessing motor dysfunction:

1. Clinical evaluation: Clinical evaluation involves a comprehensive assessment of the patient's motor function, including observation of movement, assessment of muscle tone, and evaluation of reflexes. This method can help identify movement abnormalities such as tremors, rigidity, or abnormal gait patterns.

Chapter 12: Methods for diagnosing and assessing motor dysfunction

2. Electrophysiological testing: Electrophysiological testing involves the use of electrodes to measure the electrical activity of muscles and nerves. This method can help identify neuromuscular disorders such as myopathies or neuropathies.

3. Imaging techniques: Imaging techniques such as magnetic resonance imaging (MRI) and computed tomography (CT) scans can provide detailed images of the brain and other structures involved in movement control. These methods can help identify structural abnormalities, such as tumors or lesions, that may be causing motor dysfunction.

4. Motion analysis: Motion analysis involves the use of specialized equipment to measure and analyze movement patterns. This method can provide detailed information about the kinematics and kinetics of movement, which can be useful in identifying movement abnormalities and assessing treatment outcomes.

5. Laboratory testing: Laboratory testing can help identify underlying metabolic or genetic conditions that may be contributing to motor dysfunction. For example, blood tests can help identify metabolic disorders such as mitochondrial disease, while genetic testing can identify inherited conditions such as muscular dystrophy.

6. Functional assessments: Functional assessments involve evaluating the patient's ability to perform specific tasks related to daily living or functional activities. These assessments can

help identify specific areas of impairment and guide treatment planning.

EXAMPLES

Here are some examples for each method of diagnosing and assessing motor dysfunction:

1. Clinical evaluation: Observation of tremors during rest or movement, Assessment of muscle tone, including spasticity or rigidity, Evaluation of reflexes, including deep tendon reflexes and Babinski reflex, Assessment of gait, including shuffling or dragging of feet
2. Electrophysiological testing: Electromyography (EMG) to measure muscle activity and diagnose myopathies or muscle weakness, Nerve conduction studies (NCS) to measure nerve function and diagnose neuropathies or nerve damage,
3. Imaging techniques: Magnetic resonance imaging (MRI) to detect structural abnormalities in the brain or spinal cord, Computed tomography (CT) scans to identify tumors or lesions that may be affecting movement
4. Motion analysis: Gait analysis using specialized equipment to measure walking patterns and identify gait abnormalities, Motion capture technology to measure joint angles and movement patterns during specific tasks,

Chapter 12: Methods for diagnosing and assessing motor dysfunction

5. Laboratory testing: Blood tests to diagnose metabolic disorders such as mitochondrial disease, Genetic testing to identify inherited conditions such as muscular dystrophy or Parkinson's disease
6. Functional assessments: Berg Balance Scale to assess balance and risk of falling, Timed Up and Go Test to measure the time it takes to stand up from a chair, walk a short distance, turn, and return to the chair, 9-Hole Peg Test to measure manual dexterity and upper limb function

In summary, there are several different methods for diagnosing and assessing motor dysfunction, including clinical evaluation, electrophysiological testing, imaging techniques, motion analysis, laboratory testing, and functional assessments. The choice of assessment method will depend on the specific nature of the motor dysfunction and the goals of the evaluation. A comprehensive and multidisciplinary approach to diagnosis and assessment can help ensure accurate diagnosis, effective treatment planning, and improved outcomes for patients with motor dysfunction.

NEUROIMAGING

Neuroimaging refers to the use of various imaging techniques to visualize and study the structure and function of the brain and nervous system. There are several different types of neuroimaging techniques, each with its own strengths and limitations.

Common types of neuroimaging

1. Magnetic Resonance Imaging (MRI): This technique uses a powerful magnetic field and radio waves to produce detailed images of the brain's structure and function. MRI is commonly used to diagnose and monitor a wide range of neurological disorders, including brain tumors, stroke, and multiple sclerosis.
2. Computed Tomography (CT): CT scans use X-rays to produce detailed images of the brain's structure. This technique is often used to diagnose acute neurological conditions, such as bleeding in the brain or skull fractures.
3. Positron Emission Tomography (PET): PET scans use a radioactive tracer to visualize the brain's metabolic activity. This technique is commonly used to study brain function, including cognition, emotion, and behavior.
4. Functional Magnetic Resonance Imaging (fMRI): This technique uses MRI to measure changes in blood flow to the brain, which can be used to infer patterns of brain activity associated with specific cognitive or behavioral tasks.
5. Electroencephalography (EEG): EEG measures the electrical activity of the brain using electrodes placed on the scalp. This technique is commonly used to diagnose and monitor epilepsy and other seizure disorders.

Chapter 12: Methods for diagnosing and assessing motor dysfunction

Neuroimaging plays a critical role in the diagnosis and treatment of neurological disorders, as well as in the study of normal brain function and development. It can also provide insights into the underlying mechanisms of brain disorders and guide the development of new treatments and interventions. However, neuroimaging techniques have some limitations, including cost, accessibility, and the need for specialized equipment and trained personnel.

Application of neuroimaging

Neuroimaging techniques can be used to diagnose and evaluate movement control disorders by visualizing the brain regions involved in motor function and identifying abnormalities or changes in activity patterns associated with specific movement control disorders.

For example, functional magnetic resonance imaging (fMRI) can be used to study the neural circuits involved in motor control and identify changes in brain activity associated with movement control disorders such as Parkinson's disease, dystonia, and cerebral palsy. fMRI can also be used to evaluate the effectiveness of treatments for movement control disorders and guide the development of new interventions.

Diffusion tensor imaging (DTI) is another neuroimaging technique that can be used to study the structural integrity of white matter tracts in the brain, which are critical for motor control. DTI can be used to identify changes in white matter integrity associated with movement control disorders such as multiple sclerosis, stroke, and traumatic brain injury.

Electroencephalography (EEG) and magnetoencephalography (MEG) are non-invasive neuroimaging techniques that can be used to study the electrical and magnetic activity of the brain, respectively. These techniques can be used to study the neural circuits involved in motor control and identify changes in activity patterns associated with movement control disorders.

Overall, neuroimaging techniques have the potential to provide valuable insights into the underlying mechanisms of movement control disorders, which can lead to improved diagnosis and treatment of these conditions. However, it is important to note that neuroimaging should be used in conjunction with other diagnostic methods, such as clinical evaluation and laboratory tests, to ensure accurate diagnosis and treatment.

Neuroimaging and Pakinson's disease

Neuroimaging techniques have been used to study motor dysfunction in Parkinson's disease (PD), a neurodegenerative disorder characterized by tremors, rigidity, and bradykinesia (slowness of movement). Neuroimaging has been particularly useful in understanding the changes in brain structure and function

Chapter 12: Methods for diagnosing and assessing motor dysfunction

associated with PD, and in identifying biomarkers for early diagnosis and tracking disease progression.

1. Magnetic resonance imaging (MRI) is a neuroimaging technique that has been used to study the structural changes in the brain associated with PD. Studies using MRI have identified changes in brain morphology, particularly in regions involved in motor control, such as the substantia nigra and basal ganglia. These changes can be used to differentiate between individuals with PD and healthy controls.
2. Positron emission tomography (PET) is another neuroimaging technique that has been used to study PD. PET can be used to visualize dopamine metabolism in the brain, which is altered in individuals with PD. PET can also be used to measure glucose metabolism and blood flow in regions of the brain involved in motor control, which can help identify areas of dysfunction.
3. Functional MRI (fMRI) is a neuroimaging technique that has been used to study the changes in brain activity associated with PD. Studies using fMRI have identified changes in brain activity patterns in regions involved in motor control, particularly in the early stages of PD.

Overall, neuroimaging techniques have provided valuable insights into the changes in brain structure and function associated with PD and motor dysfunction and can potentially improve early diagnosis and tracking of disease progression. However, further research is needed to fully understand the complex mechanisms underlying motor dysfunction in PD and to develop effective interventions to manage this debilitating symptom.

Neuroimaging and Alzheimer's disease

Neuroimaging techniques have been used to study the relationship between Alzheimer's disease (AD) and motor dysfunction. Motor dysfunction is a common feature of AD, characterized by impairments in gait, balance, and coordination.

1. Magnetic resonance imaging (MRI) is a neuroimaging technique that has been used to study the relationship between AD and motor dysfunction. Studies using MRI have identified changes in brain morphology, particularly in regions involved in motor control, in individuals with AD and motor dysfunction. These changes include a reduction in white matter integrity, cortical thinning, and reduced connectivity in brain regions involved in motor control.
2. Functional MRI (fMRI) is another neuroimaging technique that has been used to study the relationship between AD and motor dysfunction. fMRI can be used to study the functional connectivity of the brain and identify changes in brain activity patterns that are associated with motor dysfunction. Studies using fMRI have identified changes in brain activity patterns in regions involved in motor control, particularly in the early stages of AD.

Chapter 12: Methods for diagnosing and assessing motor dysfunction

3. Positron emission tomography (PET) is a neuroimaging technique that can be used to study the relationship between AD and motor dysfunction. PET can be used to visualize glucose metabolism in the brain, which is altered in individuals with AD and motor dysfunction. Studies using PET have identified changes in glucose metabolism in brain regions involved in motor control, suggesting a link between AD and motor dysfunction.

Overall, neuroimaging techniques have provided valuable insights into the relationship between AD and motor dysfunction, highlighting the importance of early detection and treatment of motor dysfunction in individuals with AD. However, further research is needed to fully understand the complex mechanisms underlying motor dysfunction in AD and to develop effective interventions to manage this debilitating symptom.

Neuroimaging and multiple sclerosis

Neuroimaging techniques have been used to study motor dysfunction in multiple sclerosis (MS). This chronic autoimmune disorder affects the central nervous system and can cause a wide range of symptoms, including motor dysfunction. Neuroimaging has been particularly useful in understanding the changes in brain structure and function associated with MS, and in identifying biomarkers for early diagnosis and tracking disease progression.

1. Magnetic resonance imaging (MRI) is a neuroimaging technique that has been used to study the structural changes in the brain associated with MS. Studies using MRI have identified changes in brain morphology, particularly in regions involved in motor control, such as the corticospinal tracts and cerebellum. These changes can be used to differentiate between individuals with MS and healthy controls.
2. Functional MRI (fMRI) is a neuroimaging technique that has been used to study the changes in brain activity associated with MS-related motor dysfunction. Studies using fMRI have identified changes in brain activity patterns in regions involved in motor control, particularly in the early stages of MS. fMRI can also be used to assess the effectiveness of rehabilitation interventions in improving motor function in individuals with MS.
3. Transcranial magnetic stimulation (TMS) is another neuroimaging technique that has been used to study motor dysfunction in MS. TMS can be used to measure corticospinal excitability and assess the integrity of the corticospinal tracts, which are often affected in MS-related motor dysfunction.

Overall, neuroimaging techniques have provided valuable insights into the changes in brain structure and function associated with MS and motor dysfunction, and have the potential to improve early diagnosis and tracking of disease progression. However, further

Chapter 12: Methods for diagnosing and assessing motor dysfunction

research is needed to fully understand the complex mechanisms underlying motor dysfunction in MS and to develop effective interventions to manage this debilitating symptom.

Neuroimaging and stroke

Neuroimaging techniques have been used to study motor dysfunction in stroke, a neurological disorder that occurs when the blood supply to a part of the brain is disrupted. Stroke can cause a wide range of symptoms, including motor dysfunction. Neuroimaging has been particularly useful in understanding the changes in brain structure and function associated with stroke, and in identifying biomarkers for early diagnosis and tracking of disease progression.

1. Magnetic resonance imaging (MRI) is a neuroimaging technique that has been used to study the structural changes in the brain associated with stroke. Studies using MRI have identified changes in brain morphology, particularly in regions involved in motor control, such as the corticospinal tracts and motor cortex. These changes can be used to differentiate between individuals with stroke and healthy controls, and to predict motor recovery.
2. Functional MRI (fMRI) is a neuroimaging technique that has been used to study the changes in brain activity associated with stroke-related motor dysfunction. Studies using fMRI have

identified changes in brain activity patterns in regions involved in motor control, particularly in the early stages of stroke. fMRI can also be used to assess the effectiveness of rehabilitation interventions in improving motor function in individuals with stroke.

3. Transcranial magnetic stimulation (TMS) is another neuroimaging technique that has been used to study motor dysfunction in stroke. TMS can be used to measure corticospinal excitability and assess the integrity of the corticospinal tracts, which are often affected in stroke-related motor dysfunction.

Overall, neuroimaging techniques have provided valuable insights into the changes in brain structure and function associated with stroke and motor dysfunction, and have the potential to improve early diagnosis and tracking of disease progression. However, further research is needed to fully understand the complex mechanisms underlying motor dysfunction in stroke and to develop effective interventions to manage this debilitating symptom.

Neuroimaging and spinal cord injury

Neuroimaging techniques have been used to study motor dysfunction in spinal cord injury (SCI), a neurological disorder that occurs when the spinal cord is damaged, leading to motor dysfunction. Neuroimaging has been particularly useful in

Chapter 12: Methods for diagnosing and assessing motor dysfunction

understanding the changes in brain structure and function associated with SCI, and in identifying biomarkers for early diagnosis and tracking of disease progression.

1. Magnetic resonance imaging (MRI) is a neuroimaging technique that has been used to study the structural changes in the brain and spinal cord associated with SCI. Studies using MRI have identified changes in brain and spinal cord morphology, particularly in regions involved in motor control, such as the corticospinal tracts and motor cortex. These changes can be used to differentiate between individuals with SCI and healthy controls, and to predict motor recovery.

2. Functional MRI (fMRI) is a neuroimaging technique that has been used to study the changes in brain activity associated with SCI-related motor dysfunction. Studies using fMRI have identified changes in brain activity patterns in regions involved in motor control, particularly in the early stages of SCI. fMRI can also be used to assess the effectiveness of rehabilitation interventions in improving motor function in individuals with SCI.

3. Transcranial magnetic stimulation (TMS) is another neuroimaging technique that has been used to study motor dysfunction in SCI. TMS can be used to measure corticospinal excitability and assess the integrity of the corticospinal tracts, which are often affected in SCI-related motor dysfunction.

Overall, neuroimaging techniques have provided valuable insights into the changes in brain and spinal cord structure and function associated with SCI and motor dysfunction, and have the potential to improve early diagnosis and tracking of disease progression. However, further research is needed to fully understand the complex mechanisms underlying motor dysfunction in SCI and to develop effective interventions to manage this debilitating symptom.

Neuroimaging and depression

Motor dysfunction is a common symptom of depression. Motor dysfunction can manifest in several ways, including changes in motor activity, decreased energy levels, psychomotor agitation or retardation, and changes in posture and gait. These symptoms are often associated with depression-related changes in brain function and structure, particularly in regions involved in motor control, such as the prefrontal cortex, basal ganglia, and cerebellum.

Research using neuroimaging techniques, such as functional MRI (fMRI), structural MRI, diffusion tensor imaging (DTI), and transcranial magnetic stimulation (TMS), has provided evidence of motor dysfunction in depression. Studies have identified changes in brain activity patterns and morphology in regions involved in motor control in individuals with depression, and have linked these changes to changes in motor activity and psychomotor functioning.

Chapter 12: Methods for diagnosing and assessing motor dysfunction

Therefore, motor dysfunction is a significant symptom of depression and is an important consideration in the diagnosis and management of depression.

Neuroimaging and schizophrenia

Motor dysfunction is a common symptom of schizophrenia, and neuroimaging studies have been used to investigate the neural mechanisms underlying this dysfunction. These studies have identified changes in brain activity, morphology, and connectivity in regions involved in motor control, such as the basal ganglia, thalamus, and cerebellum.

The basal ganglia is a group of subcortical structures involved in motor control, reward processing, and learning. Dysfunction in the basal ganglia has been linked to motor dysfunction in schizophrenia, particularly in the striatum and the globus pallidus. Changes in activity and connectivity of these regions have been associated with changes in motor activity, such as increased motor activation, motor disinhibition, and impaired motor coordination in individuals with schizophrenia.

The thalamus is a subcortical structure involved in sensory processing and motor control. Dysfunction in the thalamus has also been linked to motor dysfunction in schizophrenia, particularly in the ventral anterior and mediodorsal nuclei. Changes in activity and connectivity of these regions have been associated with changes in motor activity and sensory processing in individuals with schizophrenia.

The cerebellum is a region of the brain involved in motor coordination and balance. Dysfunction in the cerebellum has also been linked to motor dysfunction in schizophrenia, particularly in the posterior lobe and the vermis. Changes in activity and connectivity of these regions have been associated with changes in motor activity and sensory processing in individuals with schizophrenia.

Overall, dysfunction in these brain regions involved in motor control is thought to contribute to motor dysfunction in schizophrenia. Neuroimaging studies have helped to identify these changes and shed light on the neural mechanisms underlying motor dysfunction in schizophrenia. However, further research is needed to fully understand the nature of these changes and their relationship to other symptoms of schizophrenia.

CHAPTER 13: FUTURE DIRECTIONS IN MOTOR CONTROL RESEARCH

Motor control research has made significant progress in recent years, but there are still many questions to be answered and challenges to be addressed. Here are some emerging trends and future directions in motor control research:

1. Advances in technology: The development of new technologies, such as wearable sensors, virtual reality, and brain-computer interfaces, is opening up new possibilities for studying motor control in real-world contexts. These technologies can also be used to develop new interventions for motor dysfunction.

2. New theories and models: Emerging theories and models, such as the dynamical systems approach, are providing new insights into the mechanisms of motor control. These models emphasize the importance of the interaction between the nervous system, the environment, and the musculoskeletal system in controlling movement.

3. Neuroplasticity and motor learning: Advances in our understanding of neuroplasticity and motor learning are leading to new approaches for rehabilitating motor dysfunction. For example, non-invasive brain stimulation techniques such as transcranial magnetic stimulation (TMS) and transcranial direct current stimulation (tDCS) are being explored as potential treatments for motor disorders.

4. Multidisciplinary approaches: Motor control research is becoming increasingly multidisciplinary, with collaborations between researchers from fields such as neuroscience, engineering, and computer science. This approach can lead to new insights and innovations in the field.

5. Applications in healthcare, sport, and other fields: The insights gained from motor control research have potential applications in a wide range of fields, including healthcare, sport, and robotics. For example, the development of exoskeletons and other assistive devices can improve mobility and independence for people with motor dysfunction.

In summary, motor control research is a rapidly evolving field with exciting new developments and applications. Advances in technology, new theories and models, and multidisciplinary approaches are expanding our understanding of motor control and leading to new interventions for motor dysfunction. The potential applications of motor control research are vast, and the field is poised for continued growth and innovation in the years to come.

REFERENCES

1. Bear M., Connors B., Paradiso M. (1996). Neuroscience, Williams and Wilkins, ISBN: 0-683-00488-3
2. Brinkman, C., Porter, R., 1983. Supplementary motor area and premotor area of monkey cerebral cortex: functional organization and activities of single neurons during performance of a learned movement. Adv Neurol. 39, 393-420.
3. Brinkman, C., Porter, R., 1983. Supplementary motor area and premotor area of monkey cerebral cortex: functional organization and activities of single neurons during performance of a learned movement. Adv Neurol. 39, 393-420.
4. Fi, J.D. (1995) High-Yield Neuroanatomy, Williams and Wilkins, ISBN0-683-03248-8.
5. Keus, S. H., Munneke, M., Graziano, M., Paltamaa, J., Pelosin, E., Domingos, J., ... & Bloem, B. R. (2007). European physiotherapy guideline for Parkinson's disease. KNGF/ParkinsonNet.
6. Lang, C. E., Macdonald, J. R., Reisman, D. S., Boyd, L., Jacobson, K. T., Schindler-Ivens, S. M., ... & Wu, S. S. (2008). Observation of amounts of movement practice provided during stroke rehabilitation. Archives of physical medicine and rehabilitation, 89(4), 583-592.
7. Lundy-Ekman, L. (1998). Neuroscience: Fundamentals for Rehabilitation, W.B. Saunders Company, ISBN: 0721647170.
8. MacKay-Lyons, M., 2002. Central pattern generation of locomotion: a review of the evidence. Phys Ther. 82, 69-83.

9. MacKay-Lyons, M., 2002. Central pattern generation of locomotion: a review of the evidence. Phys Ther. 82, 69-83.

10. Mihara, M., Miyai, I., Hattori, N., Hatakenaka, M., Yagura, H., & Kawano, T. (2012). Randomized controlled trial of multisensory Stimulation-Based Intervention for motor Skill Improvement in basketball Players: A pilot study. Neurorehabilitation and Neural Repair, 26(7), 812-819.

11. Pan, C. Y. (2010). Effects of water exercise swimming program on aquatic skills and social behaviors in children with autism spectrum disorders. Autism, 14(1), 9-28.

12. Passingham, R.E., 1986. Cues for movement in monkeys (Macaca mulatta) with lesions in premotor cortex. Behav Neurosci. 100, 695-703.

13. Passingham, R.E., 1986. Cues for movement in monkeys (Macaca mulatta) with lesions in premotor cortex. Behav Neurosci. 100, 695-703.

14. Porter R. and Lemon R. (1995). Corticospinal Function and Voluntary Movement, Oxford University Press, Oxford OX26DP, ISBN0198523750

15. Reisman, D. S., Wityk, R., Silver, K., & Bastian, A. J. (2013). Split-belt treadmill training improves gait and balance in individuals with stroke. Journal of Neurologic Physical Therapy, 37(4), 185-191.

16. Rothwell J. C. (1987). Control of Human Voluntary Movement, Rothwell, John C., ISBN0-7099-2240-X.

References

17. Taylor, N. F., Dodd, K. J., & Fiers, S. (2012). The relationship between motor impairments, cognitive deficits and daily living skills in Parkinson's disease. Journal of Neural Transmission, 119(7), 743-748.
18. Van Wittenberghe, I.C., Peterson, D.C., 2022. Corticospinal Tract Lesion. In: StatPearls. Vol., ed.^eds., Treasure Island (FL).
19. Van Wittenberghe, I.C., Peterson, D.C., 2022. Corticospinal Tract Lesion. In: StatPearls. Vol., ed.^eds., Treasure Island (FL).
20. Wilson J. D., Braunwald, E. et al. (1991). Principles of Internal Medicine. New York, McGraw-Hill, Inc.
21. Zavvarian, M.M., Hong, J., Fehlings, M.G., 2020. The Functional Role of Spinal Interneurons Following Traumatic Spinal Cord Injury. Front Cell Neurosci. 14, 127.

INDEX

A muscle spindle	212
A nerve conduction velocity	248
acromioclavicular joint	392
Acromioclavicular joint dislocation	392
Akathisia	143
alcohol-induced myopathy	347
Alpha motor neuron	181
Ankle injuries	427
Ankle joint dysfunction	429
ankle region	425
Anterior dislocation of the shoulder joint	389
Apraxia	115
Arm reaching	305
Axillary nerve injury	371
Babinski sign	170
Ballism	165
basal ganglia	120
baseball finger	403
body balance	290
brachial plexus injury	366
Broca's aphasia	80
Brodmann's areas 5 and 7	83
Brodmann's areas	3
Carpal tunnel syndrome	408
central pattern generators	239
Cerebellar ataxia	303
cerebellar motor syndrome	107
cervicocollic reflex	269
Cingulate cortex	81
clasp-knife reflex	226
Cogwheel rigidity	360
Colles' fracture	398
common fibular nerve	421
Cortical columns	8
cranial nerves	269
critical component of motor learning	39
crossed extensor reflex	235
Decerebrate posture	305
Deep brain stimulation	149
Deep sensation	204
Deliberate practice	42
direct pathway	134
Directly testing muscle power	351
ecological model	18
elbow joint	393
Elbow joint dislocation	393
Electromyography	247
Endocrine myopathy	348
Environmental factors	46
Epilepsy	119
Examination of the shape and size of muscles	356
Examples of how motor learning principles	54
Extrafusal muscle fibers	214
Extrapyramidal syndrome	146
Extrinsic feedback	38

Index

factors that can influence motor skill acquisition and retention	32
Fasciculations	358
Feedback in motor learning	33
feedback to improve motor skills	35
Fine movements	307
Force	69
fracture of the distal end of the radius	397
Fracture of the neck of the femur	416
fracture of the olecranon	396
fracture of the scaphoid bone	402
Functional testing of muscle power	354
gag reflex	234
Gamma motor neurons	190
generation of spinal motor programs	238
globus pallidus	126
Golgi tendon organ	216
Golgi tendon reflex	220
Gower's sign	342
Head and neck movements	265
Hemiparesis	108
Hemiplegia	110
herniation of the nucleus pulposus	444
hierarchical model	17
hip joint	412
Hip joint dislocation	415
Hip region motor dysfunction	411
Huntington's disease	162
Hyperabduction syndrome	370
Hyperkinesia	138
Hypokinesia	142
impacted fracture of the surgical neck of the humerus	399
indirect pathway	134
Indirect testing of muscle power	353
Injuries to the infraclavicular part of the brachial plexus	369
Injury to the supraclavicular part of the brachial plexus	367
internal capsule	169
Internally guided movements	90
intracerebral hematoma	106
Intrafusal muscle fibers	213
Intrinsic feedback	36
joint	380
Joint dislocation	384
knee joint	417
Knee joint injury	423
knee region	417
Lachman's test	425
Long Thoracic Nerve Injury	372
Lower back pain	443
Lower motor neuron syndrome	257
Lower motor neurons	177
medial lemniscus pathway	206
Median nerve injury	373
Metabolic myopathy	345
motor end plate	313
motor homunculus	5
motor learning	28
Motor learning	27
Motor neuron disease	261

motor neuron pool 186
motor skill acquisition and retention 41
motor skills 29
motor unit....................................... 184
MRC scale.. 352
Muscle dysfunction......................... 333
Muscle tone 350, 359
Muscle tone changes 144
Muscle twitching............................. 210
Muscle weakness 334, 337
Myopathies 339
Myotonic dystrophy........................ 343
Nerve agents................................... 319
nerve conduction velocity............... 250
Neuroimaging 449
Orientation 72
orientation in space 298
orienting reflex 281
Paraplegia 253
Peripheral nerve injury 363
Physical therapy.............................. 147
Plasticity of the Cortical Motor Map. 74
Polymyositis.................................... 346
polysynaptic flexor reflex................ 231
posture abnormalities..................... 145
Pott's fracture 431
practice in motor skill acquisition and retention 44
Precision 70
Premotor Cortex 79
Premovement potential.................... 95
primary motor cortex lesion 111

putamen.. 124
Putamen and motor control............ 124
Quadriplegia 254
Radial Nerve Injury 375
Rapid irregular jerks 140
Raynaud's phenomenon................. 409
Ready, Set, and Go 96
Reciprocal inhibition reflex............. 227
reflex loop maintaining body posture 288
rescue reaction 294
Romberg sign.................................. 301
sciatic nerve.................................... 413
Scoliosis 289
Sensorimotor integration 23
sensory ataxia................................. 299
Sensory inputs 194
Shoulder joint dislocation............... 388
snuffbox.. 403
somatomotor cortex 59
Spastic dysarthria 111
Spike-Triggered Averaging................ 73
spinal cord 174
spinal cord injury 251
Spinal excitatory and inhibitory interneurons 192
spinocerebellar pathway 209
spinothalamic pathway 200
sprained ankle 432
stretch reflex 222
Striatum... 122
Student's elbow 406

Index

Subacromial bursitis 405
subdural hematoma 104
substantia nigra 130
Superficial sensation........................ 199
supplementary motor area................ 91
Supplementary Motor Area............... 80
Sustained muscle contraction 216
systems model................................... 18
Tardive dyskinesia 142
Tennis elbow 407
three main stages of motor learning . 30
topographic arrangement of lower
　　motor neurons............................ 179
transverse fracture of the body of the
　　humerus 400, 401
Tremor 139
Trunk movements 284
Ulnar nerve injury 376
Upper limb bursitis.......................... 404
Upper limb joint injuries 379
Upper limb motor dysfunction........ 362
Upper motor neuron syndrome 256
Upper motor neurons 176
vestibular system 295
vestibulo-ocular reflex 267
Viral myalgia.................................... 348
withdrawal reflex 231

Printed in France by Amazon
Brétigny-sur-Orge, FR